Vaccines: Are they Worth a Shot?

Andrea Grignolio

# Vaccines: Are they Worth a Shot?

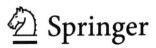 Springer

Copernicus Books is a brand of Springer

Andrea Grignolio
Unit and Museum of History of Medicine
Department of Experimental Medicine
Sapienza University of Rome
Rome, Italy

Translated by Joan Rundo
Garbagnate Milanese, Italy

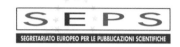

The translation of this book has been funded by SEPS SEGRETARIATO EUROPEO PER LE PUBBLICAZIONI SCIENTIFICHE, Via Val d'Aposa 7, 40123 Bologna, Italy, e-mail: seps@seps.it, www.seps.it

ISBN 978-3-319-68105-4       ISBN 978-3-319-68106-1    (eBook)
https://doi.org/10.1007/978-3-319-68106-1

Library of Congress Control Number: 2018942232

Cover illustration by Anne-Lise Boutin

Printed on acid-free paper

This Copernicus imprint is published by the registered company Springer International Publishing AG part of Springer Nature.
The registered company address is: Gewerbestrasse 11, 6330 Cham, Switzerland

*To my mother, who gave me my first immunity*

*The only true voyage of discovery, the only fountain of Eternal Youth,*
*would be not to visit strange lands,*
*but to possess other eyes.*
Marcel Proust, *The Captive*

*Liberty cannot be preserved without general knowledge among the people.*
John Adams, *Dissertation on the Canon and Feudal Law*

*Truth, the harsh truth.*
Stendhal, *The red and the black*

# Foreword

Vaccines have led us out of the Age of Darkness into the Age of Enlightenment. Because of vaccines, children no longer have to routinely suffer diseases like meningitis, hepatitis, pneumonia, and sepsis and a variety of other potentially fatal infections. Unfortunately, vaccines have now become a victim of their own success. Young parents today don't see many of these diseases; they didn't grow up with them. For these parents, the promise of vaccines is not nearly as compelling as it was decades ago.

Further, we have moved from an era where scientific illiteracy has been replaced by scientific denialism. People simply declare their own "truths" no matter how much information is available to refute them. Perhaps worst of all, many people have become afraid of scientific advances, worried that we have stepped beyond our bounds and that we are doing more harm than good. "We have guided missiles but misguided men," said Martin Luther King, Jr.

Into the fray steps Andrea Grignolio. Unlike previous books on the subject, *Vaccines: Are they Worth a Shot?* takes a broad overview of the problem. Not only does Grignolio address the history of the anti-vaccine movement starting with humankind's first vaccine, smallpox; he also examines the political, evolutionary, sociological, and media influences that impact how we perceive vaccines. Perhaps most interesting, Grignolio examines changes in the doctor–patient relationship, why as a society we have moved from skepticism to cynicism, how we perceive risk, and how we reason.

*Vaccines: Are they Worth a Shot?* also offers a way out: a practical guide for how to separate good information from bad information. As more and more parents choose not to vaccinate their children and as the number of preventable outbreaks of serious infectious diseases increases, Grignolio's book is a timely and important addition to a problem that can no longer be ignored.

Much is at stake.

Division of Infectious Diseases,                                    Paul A. Offit
Vaccine Education Center,
The Children's Hospital of Philadelphia,
Philadelphia, PA, USA

Maurice R. Hilleman Professor of Vaccinology,
Perelman School of Medicine at the
University of Pennsylvania,
Philadelphia, PA, USA

# Contents

# 1

## Who Is Afraid of Vaccines?

## The 1980s: When the Decline Started

The history of anti-vaccination movements is long and instructive. We can trace its beginnings back to late eighteenth century England and the practice of vaccinating against smallpox. From a historical point of view, we cannot say that opposition to vaccinations is anything new; what is new today is the increasingly large number of people involved and their social status. In addition, for the first time, we are seeing a decline in the vaccinal coverage of the population after two centuries of slow but inevitable advances: we are consequently seeing something very different from the opposition to vaccination in the past by some marginal groups.

We are losing what is known as *herd immunity* (also called *community, group or flock immunity*) thanks to which infectious diseases do not spread in a population if a certain percentage of individuals (which varies from 85% to 95%, depending on the contagiousness of the disease) has been vaccinated; this is a central concept which we will come back to several times. This drop in the threshold of vaccination coverage is not easy to explain, but history, as always, can help us understand.

In the past, vaccination was something unknown to which the population, with a very low rate of literacy, was subjected. They accepted a procedure which to their eyes could not fail to appear counter-productive: inoculating an infectious agent into people to make them immune towards probable future epidemics. Yet, in the nineteenth century, this practice successfully spread from London, with the preventive inoculation of attenuated smallpox, to

A. Grignolio, *Vaccines: Are they Worth a Shot?*, https://doi.org/10.1007/978-3-319-68106-1_1

Europe and the United States. This was thanks to (as we will see in Chap. 5) the active participation of wide sectors of the cultivated population and above all, of the aristocracy, obviously together with other factors such as literacy and the promotion of public hygiene.

After almost two centuries of fighting smallpox, the first vaccinations against rabies, anthrax, diphtheria and cholera arrived at the end of the nineteenth century, but there was a real explosion in vaccinations in the twentieth century, which we can define the century of vaccinations. Diseases with a high mortality rate (with names that are still terrifying today: plague, tuberculosis, typhus, yellow fever and smallpox), which had claimed the lives of millions of people, started to recede for the first time, thanks to the vaccinal prophylaxis. Together with smallpox, the eradication of poliomyelitis—after peak diffusion had been reached in the mid-1950s in the United States and in Europe—was an unprecedented success: in December 1979, the World Health Organization (from now on WHO) announced the global disappearance of smallpox, while the last cases were registered in 1979 and 1982, respectively, in the USA and in Italy.

The 1970s were probably the highest point of the success and involvement of the population, as it was also the decade in which the MPR vaccine (also known as MMR vaccine) was introduced for measles, parotitis (commonly known as *mumps*) and rubella (or German measles). These are diseases which usually affect children by 5 years of age and which, contrary to popular belief, have a mortality rate that is anything but negligible.

In the early 1980s, nobody could have imagined that from then onwards there would have been a growing lack of confidence in vaccinations, with mistrust spreading above all in the most educated and affluent sectors of the population. Today, several Western countries have whole regions under the threshold of safety for diseases such as measles, diphtheria, German measles, mumps, whooping cough and some forms of meningitis. Why, then, from the 1980s onwards, after two centuries of success after terrible infectious diseases, have parents shown an irrational attitude towards vaccinations, refusing this treatment for their children? Besides, these parents belong to advanced democracies, have a good level of education and a good or high social and economic status—all characteristics which usually are correlated with longevity and an efficient relationship with the best medical and health behaviour.

The reasons for this inversion of trend will be discussed in detail in this book, but here we can mention the main ones, focusing our attention on the parents of children of vaccination age (3 months–15 years). There are fundamentally three reasons: neurocognitive, social and evolutionary. Let's start with the first ones.

# A Neurocognitive Explanation: Education and Risk

Vaccinations are a prophylaxis (from the ancient Greek *prophylaxis*, meaning "I prevent", "I preserve", from which *prophylactic*, meaning the male prophylactic against sexually transmittable diseases, also comes), a preventive treatment made up of rules and measures which have to be adopted collectively or by individuals, to offer protection from the spread of specific diseases, both infectious and not. Unlike other prophylactic practices, which come within the rules of preventive medicine, vaccination is fairly counter-intuitive and, therefore, particularly difficult to understand. Let's take the example of two well-known cases such as oral hygiene or asbestos. Cleaning your teeth every day with a toothbrush and fluoride toothpaste is part of the dental prophylaxis to keep bacterial plaque and tartar under control and to remove residues of food and sugar. Oral hygiene is something that can be perceived, as well as an aesthetic and even cultural question. In addition, anyone who neglects their oral hygiene is headed towards a progressive inflammation of the gums and, in the end, painful toothache, a gradual and tangible pathological process. Less evident, but again easily understandable, are the reasons for the prophylaxis of workplaces full of dust or particles that are dangerous for human health. These are cases in which high rates of diseases from intoxication are known, especially in the community of workers of certain chemical companies. Whereas in the case of oral hygiene, the agent to be protected from is invisible to the naked eye and the onset of pathologies is gradual; the prophylaxis for asbestos consists of perceivable procedures, such as decontaminating workplaces, limiting the production and spread of the harmful dusts and, lastly, reducing human exposure through masks, overalls and breathing apparatus etc. The case of vaccinations, i.e. the prophylaxis against infectious diseases through inoculation of the pathogenic agent for preventive purposes (we will see that there are also therapeutic vaccines), is much more complicated to understand and accept. We have to reflect on the fact that paediatric vaccinations are a pharmacological treatment which is applied not only to adults in unhealthy contexts but also to children who live in (apparently) safe environments: this is a substantial difference. To understand it, it is sufficient to examine the cases of children affected by severe pathologies caused by cancer, by autoimmune diseases or by major physical traumas: their parents show almost no resistance to therapeutic or analgesic drugs, which are by no means free of possible side effects. When it is a question of dealing with a disease or physical pain, deciding on the risks/benefits of a drug is made on fairly rational and pragmatic bases. Unlike other drugs or medication given in illness, the vaccine has to be administered to a child in a good state of health. Those who do not know that the production processes are controlled, safe and certified by continuous studies and international bodies, also see it as a pharmacological treatment with a potential risk, coming from the inoculation of a pathogenic agent with attenuated virulence (as we will see better in Chap. 5). "Live attenuated", however, is only one of the possible ways of producing vaccines: there are also "inactivated" vaccines (in which the infectious agent has been killed), the ones against pathogenic subunits and toxins, and, lastly, those constructed with molecular strategies from genetic material or protein portions of the pathogenic agent. It is not always easy for a parent to accept that a pathogenic agent, or a derivative of it, is injected into their child's blood purely for prevention. This first reason for refusal by parents is not to be attributed only to the generations that lived in the 1980s but we will see how in actual fact, from that period onwards, TV and the press started to circulate erroneous beliefs and stories breeding anxiety about vaccines, increasing in parents the perception of the risks of vaccination rather than of the diseases from which they offer protection.

The very concept of prevention is actually a source of great confusion and refers to a second problem in the neurocognitive context: today, subjects are vaccinated in the presence of a risk that cannot be seen, but only imagined. Luckily, the infectious diseases have virtually disappeared, but the microbes that cause them are still here. From the 1980s, the disappearance from the streets in our cities of semi-paralysed invalids with poliomyelitis, people with tuberculosis exhausted by consumption or people disfigured by smallpox also meant the loss of effective social alarms and of useful evidence of the perception of the collective risk. In this case too, not all parents are willing to rationally face a risk which is real but not visible. It is not infrequent to hear that in Western countries, "severe" infectious diseases have now disappeared or that "minor" diseases such as measles, diphtheria, chicken pox, whooping cough and tetanus can be naturally contracted by unvaccinated children without risks. In actual fact, both the pathogenicity (the capacity of a microorganism to inflict damage on its host and give disease) and the contagiousness (the capacity of a microorganism to naturally transmit from an infected animal, even though a healthy carrier, to a receptive one) of infectious diseases has been reduced precisely thanks to the spread of vaccines (again see Chap. 5). For this reason, compared to 30 years ago, infectious paediatric diseases today are less aggressive and common; proof of this is that the recent drop in vaccinal coverage has inverted this trend, making very virulent strains re-emerge which have caused several deaths. Only to mention some data from recent months and relative to geographical areas close to us, in 2015, several unvaccinated children lost their lives, in particular: in March a 4-year-old girl at the Bambin Gesù Hospital in Rome died of measles; in October a baby of only 1 month—the victim of the lack of herd immunity as it was without vaccinal cover being of pre-vaccinal age—in Bologna, from whooping cough; in June a 6-year-old girl in Spain died of diphtheria (making an alarming return 30 years after it had disappeared in 1986!); and, lastly, an outbreak of meningitis in Tuscany led to the deaths of seven people. This epidemic in only the first 3 months of 2016 had already killed four people, again in Tuscany, and between the end of 2015 and the early months of 2016, a health emergency against measles had already been recorded in Milan: 50 cases and several admissions to hospital. Lastly, in March 2016, a Dutch girl aged three, who had not been vaccinated, died of diphtheria at the hospital of Antwerp, without the doctors being able to find the drugs necessary (diphtheria antitoxin) against this infectious disease, erroneously believed to have been eradicated.

There is also a third, fairly complicated reasoning which escapes the parents who oppose vaccinations: it is the idea that their child can avoid being vaccinated in consideration of the fact that all the others have already been made immune by the vaccinations. This reasoning is wrong and morally questionable, because it ignores a central element. Vaccinations work as a collective phenomenon, not an individual one. When viruses and bacteria enter an individual, they multiply very quickly, and in doing so change significantly, modifying their conformation and ending up by differentiating themselves from the initial standard strains on which the vaccines have been formulated. A little like in the game of Chinese whispers, when a sentence sent to the first member of a group reaches the last one saying completely different things, from one infection to the next, the virus modifies its characteristics becoming difficult to identify. This means that if in a class there are children who have not been vaccinated, not only, as is obvious, are they themselves the most in danger if an infectious agent is in circulation but less intuitively, they also represent the host organisms (called *reservoir*) in which the pathogens develop and are diversified, thus gaining the ability to infect their vaccinated classmates, whose immune system does not recognize the changed forms: this is the mechanism on which herd immunity is based. If 95% of the pupils in a class are vaccinated (let's say 19 out of 20 children), then it is improbable that the virus can spread, also because if an unvaccinated child were to be infected, the number of transformations (mutations) of the incubated pathogen would not be such as to dramatically change its characteristics: it will try to infect the other classmates, but with all probability the contagion will stop because the immune system of the vaccinated children will identify it and the antibodies will eliminate them, recognizing them as a "brother" of the standard pathogen inoculated with the vaccine. If, however, there are two children (90% coverage) in the class without vaccinal cover, then it is likely that the pathogenic agent can infect the second individual as well and in the two passages it would succeed in being sufficiently transformed so not to be recognized by the antibodies of the vaccinated classmates, who would therefore be infected. This is why it is nonsense not to vaccinate one's children thinking that they can benefit from the coverage of the others, and the threshold of 95% is too high for someone to arbitrarily allow themselves the luxury of not respecting this rule of common protection. In addition, there is an ethical consideration that recalls some phenomena of biological parasitism: it is incorrect to enjoy the social benefits of immunization without taking on the risks as well, even though very rare, of the allergic reactions sometimes caused by vaccinations. Although the percentage of adverse effects from vaccinations is the lowest of all the drugs available today—about one case out of a million (as I will show in Chap. 5)—this risk has to be shared by the whole population. Only the individuals of a pre-vaccinal age, those who have immune deficiencies, such as for example cancer patients, those who are affected by autoimmune diseases or patients who have undergone transplants are morally exempt and they are exactly the people who are in extreme need of the coverage of the collective herd in order to survive.

These three reasons can all be traced back to a mistaken perception of the risks/benefits ratio, which will be discussed in greater depth below (in the paragraph on late fertility in this chapter and in Chap. 6). In actual fact, the ability to evaluate the balance between risks and benefits is central not only in vaccinations but in the whole of medicine, and it is also particularly significant in the world of finance, in many political decisions and in many other areas of today's knowledge society. Today, there is an over-production of data, personal computers are commonplace and access to the Internet is easy. This means that complex data which were once restricted to experts—such as scientific articles or reports on drug safety or the adverse effects of drugs and vaccinations in the phase of post-marketing control—are now within reach of people who do not have the knowledge required to contextualize and interpret it. They then repost this information in an alarming way on the Internet, where it can be uncritically reposted. We are not talking here about the creation of pseudo-scientific hoaxes, a very central theme in vaccines, to which a whole chapter (Chap. 3) will be devoted, but simply about the fact that, due to an apparent paradox, having more information does not always lead to making the correct decisions, especially if these entail a risk (Covello et al. 1986; Covello and Sandman 2001; Morini 2014; Gigerenzer 2015). The reasons for this behaviour have become clear in very recent years thanks to a series of interesting publications on neuroscience, behavioural economy and cognitive psychology and which explain how the human mind has evolved in a past biological context which today makes it unsuitable to assess long-term predictions, calculate uncertainties and above all, risks. This "bounded rationality" (a topic which led to the Israeli psychologist Daniel Kahneman being awarded a Nobel Prize in 2002) concerns all the sectors of the population, as it is an evolutionary trait of the human species (Kahneman 2012). If, however, we ask which sectors of the population are most subject to information overload and the assessment of risk in a medical context, we can understand immediately that it is the most affluent and educated ones. This is why the social reasons and lastly the evolutionary ones, of the refusal of vaccination, have to be analysed.

Let's take one small step backwards. In the past few decades, there has been great insistence on the fact that it was the so-called high sector of the population that had the best understanding of hygiene and health practices and the most efficient access to medical and pharmacological therapies and therefore was also the one with the greatest longevity. Therefore, in the population, a good education and economic possibilities correspond on average to a better state of health. All this is statistically valid, although unfair, as shown by the very name of the disciplinary context that deals with this: *health inequalities* (Crimmins et al. 2011; Grignolio and Franceschi 2012; Neumayer and Plumper 2015).[1] How can it be explained, then, that in the same segment of the population this ratio can be inverted, from positive to negative, precisely when we are talking about vaccines? To simplify, we could say that the ratio is inverted only when a potential risk is involved together with multiple contradictory pieces of information. This is effectively the case of vaccines (Casiday 2007) and a few other topics linked to technological and biomedical innovations, such as some advanced therapeutic treatments (Cassell et al. 2006), global warming (Kahan et al. 2012), nanotechnologies (Kahan et al. 2009) and genetically modified organisms (Finucane 2002; Blancke et al. 2015).

Is it more sensible to offer children immunity from potentially lethal disease or leave them uncovered out of fear of a severe allergic reaction that appears following one vaccination out of a million? Why are those who fear these very rare adverse events linked to vaccinations willing, to relieve negligible malaises, to ignore the risks (hundreds of times greater) of severe side effects caused by common anti-inflammatories and aspirin? Why don't the more radical parents who refuse vaccinations out of fear of autism change

---

[1] See the website and manual of the WHO (http://tinyurl.com/jysh983I) and the one promoted by the European Community through EuroHealthNet (http://eurohealthnet.eu/).

their minds even if they are shown evidence and clear data that show the extraneousness of that disease to vaccination? All this happens because during the decision-making processes in which risk, uncertainty, probability and long-term forecasts appear, the brain of *Homo sapiens* does not make rational decisions, having had an evolutionary story that has not selected it to face up to these topics, which have emerged in too recent a past. Today we know, for example, that our brain tends to remember and give greater importance to the information that suggests a high risk, even if it is statistically insignificant, whilst it tends to underestimate the benefits or low-risk information, even though offered by institutional bodies (Viscusi 1997; Kahan 2014). This is exactly what happens in the brain of a parent when they come face to face with the decision-making processes that concern vaccinations for their children. This also explains why the so-called high sector of the population is particularly critical or doubtful with regard to vaccines: it is the most informed part of the population and is, therefore, exposed to information on the calculation of risks and benefits (Ogilvie et al. 2010; Anderberg et al. 2011; Brown et al. 2012). These parents have fairly elaborate cultural instruments, are mainly university graduates who, before vaccinating their children, decide to read up on the subject, often on the Internet and, coming up against "contradictory opinions" on vaccinations, end up by hesitating or even rejecting them.

The data of some Western countries available on these parents are fairly coherent, let's have a look at them.

43.55% of US citizens use the Internet to look for health information (Amante et al. 2015). On vaccines, in particular, a study of 2015 shows that it is "young, more educated parents and who oppose the requests of vaccinations for school admission who, with respect to pro-vaccination parents, use the Internet more as a source of information on vaccinations"; they are also the parents who have a low perception of the safety and efficacy of vaccines and, naturally, have the greatest rate of vaccinal exemption for non-medical reasons, or they use personal/philosophical or religious reasons. These parents who obtain "vaccinal information on the Internet are young, have a high educational qualification and a high family income" and coincide with that part of the population who "has not subjected their children to any of the routine school vaccinations" (Jones et al. 2012; Smith et al. 2004). As in other countries, we will see shortly that the vast majority of parents, still in the USA, deem that vaccinations are safe and 83% think even what on the Internet is accused of causing autism, i.e. the MMR vaccine, is safe, even though there is a consistent and growing 9% of parents who deem the vaccines unsafe, with an additional 7% saying they don't know or are undecided. A comparative analysis between 2006 and 2013 reveals that in this period of time, the US paediatricians who reported documentation of the refusal of vaccinations by parents went from 74.5% to 87.0% and as a consequence their termination of the care relationship with the anti-vaccination families went from 6.1% to 11.7% (Hough-Telford et al. 2016; O'Leary et al. 2015), 68% (in 2009 69%) deem that the vaccines ought to be required for all children (the Hispanic minority is more favourable compared to non-Hispanic whites) while 30% (which becomes 41% of young parents between 18 and 29 years of age) deem that it has to remain a free choice of the family. With respect to the parents' decision on vaccinations, while in 2009 there was no difference regarding the political affiliation, in the 2015 surveys, Republicans were more in favour (34%) than Democrats (22%) (Anderson 2015) who appeared less inclined to allow exemption.

One study reveals that in Canada, where 57% of the interviewees said they went online (Google, social media, websites, etc.) for health information, in the case of an infectious onset of diseases preventable by vaccination, 335 would look for information on the Internet and 145 on the social media, and only 5% would use scientific sources (journals). The information obtained on the Internet influences the users in a contradictory way because although the majority (92%) believes that vaccines are safe and effective and only 6% decide not to vaccinate their children, no less than 28% of the interviewees believe that vaccines are related to autism, 27% that they can cause serious illnesses and 33% that compulsory vaccination is orchestrated by the pharmaceutical industries: these are typical arguments that come from the "rhetorical artillery of the anti-vaccine movements", increasing the share of parents hesitating over-vaccinations up to 35% (Greenberg et al. 2017).

In Australia, the Internet is the third source of health information, followed by 27% of citizens, preceded by the health authorities and institutions (28%) and the general physician (83%), who, although resisting as the most influential figure (8.37 out of 10) in the health context, is closely followed by the growing influence of the specialist (7.89 out of 10) and especially by those who practise "alternative treatments" (7.81 out of 10). The enquiry sample confirms that the Internet is followed as a source of health information far more (52%) by the groups that do not trust the classic health services compared (24%) to those on the other hand that do trust them, and while only 17% of the pro-vaccine people went on the Internet to look for the relative information, 50% of the anti-vaccine people used the web for information. The population that uses the web most for information tends to be young and also often trusts sectarian information, i.e. from family and friends. Even though 92% declare that they agree in full with vaccinating their children,

53% state that they have some problems with vaccines and 8% delay or refuse them (Chow et al. 2017).

In Italy, a 2014 analysis by the Censis (Centre for Social Investment Studies)[2] on the relationship between parents and vaccinations indicates that 7.8 % of parents "decide not to vaccinate their child on the basis of information found on the Internet". This percentage becomes even higher if the educational qualification is analysed, as 10% have a degree or higher and 9% a high school diploma or professional qualification, while parents with a middle school diploma are absent (0.0%); the less educated portion of the population is, therefore, exempt from the disinformation delivered by the Internet and when they do use it, they tend to consult the institutional websites (Ministry of Health and Higher Institute of Health). Although for 55% of parents, the most consulted source is the paediatrician; those who go to the Internet to find information on health form 32% of the sample. Apart from 40% who refer to official information on institutional sites, where obviously the data are reliable and vaccinations are recommended, the remaining 27% go to forums and blogs and 16% to the social networks (Facebook, Twitter, Instagram, Google+, MySpace) where opinions and beliefs against vaccinations flourish: 61.7% of parents who consult the Internet believe that vaccinations can be the cause of severe diseases like autism. This misleading information makes 47% of them focus their research on the risks of vaccines (against 27% who highlight the advantages) and 20% who concentrate on the stories of cases that have experienced negative effects due to vaccines. Overall, the Censis report reminds us, "78% is the percentage of interviewees who have surfed the Internet with the intention of finding information on vaccines and judges this information negative", and the opinions of the parents who consult social networks, forums and blogs to find information on vaccination reveals that more than half of them (39.7%) judge it "contrary to the MMR vaccination" with a tendency to perceive online information negatively more common "amongst parents with intermediate and high educational qualifications" (Ruiz and Bell 2014).

The vaccine most affected by these fears is, as mentioned, the trivalent MMR which protects against measles, mumps and rubella. Developed in 1971 by the American microbiologist Maurice Hilleman—who in his career developed about forty vaccines, and to whom is attributed the merit of having saved

---

[2] Censis. Cultura della vaccinazione in Italia: un'indagine sui genitori, ottobre 2014. The sample of the survey is made up of parents between 18 and 55 with children aged between 0 and 15 (the age group of the paediatrical vaccinal calendars). The percentages of this paragraph, when not indicated otherwise, are from this source: http://tinyurl.com/hcjdzqc

more lives than any other scientist of the twentieth century (Dove 2005)—in 1998 the MMR vaccine was unjustly accused of causing autism by an English doctor, Andrew Wakefield. From then on, the belief that there existed a relationship between autism and vaccines spread virally in the media and this belief was dented (we will see why in Chap. 3) neither by the data from the research of international committees made up of independent experts (and therefore without any conflicts of interest with the multinational corporations) which regularly prove the falsity of this relation nor by the fact that in 2004 it was shown how the accusation of creating autism had been deliberately constructed by Wakefield: he had altered the data in order to promote an alternate treatment of his own (see the paragraph, again in Chap. 3, on false or manipulated reconstructions, in particular in the case of autism). Due to an unforeseeable domino effect, that the economists call *spillover*, the fears, initially concentrated on the MMR vaccine, ended up in a few years involving various other vaccines, from the ones for children to the flu vaccines prescribed for the elderly and the vaccine for *papilloma virus* (HPV) for teenagers (Anderberg et al. 2011; Ogilvie et al. 2010), to the point that today 62% of parents fear that vaccines can cause diseases such as autism.

## Social Changes: The Doctor–Patient Relationship

Alongside these neurocognitive reasons, there are also changes which we could define social, such as for example the changed doctor–patient relationship. For thousands of years, the authority of the figure of the healer played a central role in human societies, with the key role of the mediator of pain and illness. Starting from the first forms of civilization, the figure of the shaman, of the healer priest (interpreter of oracles) and lastly of the doctor have followed on one another. Without efficient treatment instruments until the mid-nineteenth century, with the advent of pharmacology, these figures placed their capacity of treatment in the therapeutic alliance with the patient: a process made up of rites, words and above all suggestion based on trust, admiration and the hope inspired by the doctor. All this was made possible by the neurophysiological mechanisms which are at the base of the placebo effect, i.e. the capacity of auto-suggestion which, in response to the expectations of treatment, can put into circulation a series of endorphins—hormones, mediators and real natural drugs such as serotonin—capable of modulating the perception of pain, the cardiovascular response and the immune reaction (Benedetti 2014). This neurophysiological response, still potentially active in the doctor–patient relationship, helps to face a disease that is not treated with medicine while, if a pharmacological therapy is present, it helps the effects by increasing the performance by as much as 30%. In essence, a participating and empathic doctor triggers off in the patient this response and therefore treats better than a hasty doctor, but for this to be possible, the patient also has to place trust in the doctor and recognize his/her authority. This relationship of trust, which remained unchanged for centuries, started to fracture in the twentieth century, and today the authority of the doctor is seen almost with suspicion. In specialized literature, the wrong attitude of the doctor who takes decisions autonomously, without offering the patient a series of explanations and alternatives (when they exist) so that the patient can choose his/her own course of treatment, is defined as *paternalism*. This revolution in the doctor–patient relationship is due without any doubt to the increase in literacy, thanks to which patients are more aware and willing to play an active part in the therapies, as well as the availability of medical information on the Internet, once the prerogative only of experts. Alongside these explanations which concern the patient, some traumatic events which have broken down the authority and the *super partes* role of the doctor also have to be mentioned: the case of the ignoble experiments perpetrated by the Nazi doctors in concentration camps using prisoners as guinea pigs, or the experiments on the rural community of African Americans in Alabama, in which the natural progression of syphilis, intentionally not treated, was studied, by the U.S. Public Health Service between 1932 and 1972—it is following these events that *informed consent* came about, that all of us sign today before any medical-health treatment, precisely to avoid possible new abuses. At the end of the 1980s, the epidemic caused by the HIV virus further eroded the authority of doctors and fuelled the drive towards patient autonomy thanks to a group of activists who, in the community of AIDS victims of San Francisco, succeeded in imposing on the scientific community the deregulation of some experimental therapies (Emanuel and Grady 2008).

Today this refusal of paternalism has gone beyond the limits, in some cases risking endangering public health. If on the one hand, it is correct to involve patients in therapeutic decisions, on the other hand they cannot and can never replace the doctor and decide what is and what is not a scientifically proven therapy—but this is exactly what is happening. It is not infrequent to see television programmes in which representatives of the scientific community who have dedicated their lives to collecting data and evidence in favour of a therapy of proven efficacy, are confronted by subjects, often charlatans and conspiracy theorists, who maintain the validity of "alternative treatments". In this sense, it is sufficient to recall, although in their diversity, some traumatic events which have attracted the attention of media and politics.

In recent years in the United States, there have been a number of cases in which skilful charlatans have succeeded in gaining extensive visibility in television and on the Internet, dispensing false hopes for the health of citizens. They can be divided into two different categories of risk. The relatively less severe cases concern at least four well-known figures who sell or recommend products for the diet and well-being. Whether they are heart surgeons, osteopaths, "experts" on nutrition or toxic particles, they are media stars who offer, against payment, products or nutritional advice against ingredients deemed allergenic or carcinogenic, against the use of drinking water with added fluoride, microwave ovens and vaccinations (deemed harmful because they can cause autism or because they are rich in toxic metals) or by declaring they are in favour of the wildest conspiracy theories such as those on chemical trails or those that deny the relationship between AIDS and HIV, with a general critical attitude towards conventional medicine and pharmacological therapies, attacked because they are "chemical" and a preference for "alternative" treatments because they are deemed "natural". The most severe cases, on the other hand, concern the fake cancer or stem cell treatments maintained by ferocious charlatans. These supposed "therapies" are particularly odious because they have to do with terminally ill patients, with people and families weakened by suffering, willing to give in to irrationality and false hopes, but also because, having to do with pain, they often attract the media and not infrequently they find support in some VIP who is naïve or, worse, in search of visibility. Regarding cancer, a recent and famous case concerns a charlatan, who defined himself a "cancer coach" and, to promote his ranting, produced several books and especially a documentary in a dozen episodes on the single cases of patients who declare they fell ill due to chemotherapy and ensure, in front of television cameras, without showing any documentary scientific evidence, that they are better thanks to a treatment based on natural extracts. Following these episodes, several patients, including some who were young, decided to stop scientifically validated treatments which in certain cases, as in some infantile leukaemia, have margins of success around 90%: taking them off chemotherapy is effectively equivalent to a death sentence.[3] These fake anti-cancer drugs are so widespread that in 2017 the FDA made an announcement to American consumers where the keywords on the labels of the packaging are listed so that they can be easily identified as "cruel deceit" and avoided as a fraudulent

---

[3] Hall H., *"The Truth About Cancer" Series Is Untruthful About Cancer*, Science-Based Medicine, Nov. 17, 2015: https://goo.gl/J8p776; David Gorski (Orac), *Insolence. Another cancer quack dies. . . of cancer*, ScienceBlogs, Jul. 15, 2016: https://goo.gl/GxwJSE

product.[4] There has also been a great deal of media clamour on stem cell therapy in recent years. In the USA, as in the rest of the world, various fake stem cell clinics (about 200) are flourishing which offer preparations "based on stem cells", a sort of new "snake oil" without any respect for the regulatory rules imposed by the FDA. These laboratories were the starting base for a group of four charlatans, then criminally prosecuted (with 39 charges) who between 2007 and 2010 were able to earn $1.5 million from people who suffered from a wide variety of diseases (amyotrophic lateral sclerosis, Parkinson's disease, muscular dystrophy, cancer), by injecting them with this "miraculous preparation of stem cells" in a series of four infusions. The case of a doctor (who in 2005 lost his licence) is famous, because he was the subject of a television investigation: with his personal potion based on stem cells he maintained that he could "cure" 70 diseases at a price which ranged from $2500 to $20,000, even offering diagnoses and therapies by conference call.[5] Another "network of clinics" offer on the web therapies for at least two dozen diseases, the most requested of which included supposed treatments for heart failure, pulmonary diseases, glaucoma and macular degeneration linked to age—on the last-named, a 2017 report by the authoritative *New England Journal of Medicine* denounced several cases of severe permanent damage, including three women who lost their sight (Kuriyan et al. 2017). Alongside these two groups of charlatans, distinguished by their gravity and impact on the lives of the patients, stem cells also offer a middle path between stem cell therapy and nutritional or naturalist advice: the use of stem cells for aesthetic purposes. A number of Californian "clinics" have recently been the subject of great media clamour as they offered a treatment, at the cost of about $9000 for liposuction based on stem cells, in which adipose tissue is extracted from the patient, and the stem cells allegedly isolated from this tissue and then reinfused in the patient together with other enzymes. These treatments are difficult to prosecute in the USA because they fall into a regulatory loophole not covered by the supervisory body, the FDA, which does not recognize them as drugs but as injections. These treatments are considered "minimally manipulated biological products" where the biological material is extracted and reinserted in the patient in the same session, with low risks of contamination and of diffusion of any infectious material. Some of these clinics state on their website that they also offer, alongside the aesthetic operations,

---

[4] U.S. Food & Drug Administration (FDA), For Consumers, *Products Claiming to "Cure" Cancer Are a Cruel Deception*, Apr. 25, 2017: https://goo.gl/Qi34iv

[5] Stem Cells Portal. The Stem Cells and Regenerative Medicine Online Community, *Stem Cells Fraud Scheme in U.S. Leads to Arrests*, January 18, 2012: https://goo.gl/TqrCAA

treatments for orthopaedic problems, arthritis and joint pain. As is often the case, the area of aesthetic medicine often converges into treatments for well-being and both in New York and Los Angeles products for the skin and wrinkles "based on stem cells" are becoming popular. Scientists warn keeping away but sometimes a celebrity only has to say that she uses these products for them to become a credible and effective treatment.[6]

In the United Kingdom, the most important fraud concerns the fake study by Wakefield (see Chap. 3 for further details) who in 1998 accused the MMR vaccine of causing autism. This false information spread thanks to a series of documentaries and was then relaunched virally on the web. If other countries, influenced by this fraud, show fears for the MMR vaccine, it was in England that it created the greatest scepticism in parents, who quote the Wakefield affair as the cause of their critical attitude towards vaccinations (Casiday et al. 2006; Yaqub et al. 2014). A comparative study on the hesitation towards parents in India, Pakistan, Nigeria, Georgia and the United Kingdom showed that the last-named country had the highest rate of hesitant parents, 24.5%, of whom one-quarter, 27.1%, expressed a radical opposition to vaccinating their children (Larson and Schulz 2015). The consequence was that in the United Kingdom after 1998 the MMR vaccine significantly fell below the standard of 95% of coverage of the population required by WHO: between 2006 and 2009, the percentage remained around 85% and it was not until 2014 that the level of coverage returned to pre-Wakefield levels, recording 92.3% in 2016–2016 (Brown et al. 2012; Yaqub et al. 2014).[7]

Germany is not exempt from biomedical fraud either. In 2007, two clinics were opened, first in Cologne and then in Düsseldorf, (XCell-Centers), where presumed stem cell therapies were offered to treat a wide range of neurodegenerative diseases: traumas to the spine, various neuropathies, cerebral paralysis, arthritis, cardiovascular diseases and incontinence. Stem cells from the marrow were extracted from the patients, who had paid on average 25,000 €, and it was then reinfused in the brain, in the spine or in the blood, depending on the pathology. In 2010, the centre was closed after a child of ten suffered severe permanent damage following a badly conducted operation and after a child of 18 months died due to an injection of stem cells in the brain. The

---

[6] Jabr, F., *In the Flesh: The Embedded Dangers of Untested Stem Cell Cosmetics. Unapproved procedures and skin care products endanger consumers and clinical research*, "Scientific American", Dec. 17, 2012: https://goo.gl/UtQjMs; Engel M., Kuntzman G., *Celebs' stem cell facial treatments include sheep placenta, others get human cells*, "New York Daily News", Mar. 27, 2015: https://goo.gl/fKyg8h; MCFarling U.L., *FDA moves to crack down on unproven stem cell therapies*, "STAT", Feb. 8, 2016: https://goo.gl/pHc353

[7] NHS Immunisation Statistics. England, 2015–16. Sept. 22, 2016: http://content.digital.nhs.uk/catalogue/PUB21651/nhs-imms-stat-eng-2015-16-rep.pdf

international resonance on the affair fuelled by an investigation by the British newspaper *The Sunday Telegraph* made the German Parliament rapidly update the regulation on the use of stem cells in order to avoid similar new frauds (Mummery et al. 2014). The most famous of the charlatans on "alternative therapies" for cancer also came from Germany, namely Ryke Geerd Hamer, father of New German Medicine. Based on a series of fantasies, that his inventor defined "the five fundamental biological laws," according to the so-called Hamer method cancer was the result of a trauma or a psychological conflict. When this conflict has been solved, the cancer regresses. After the first deaths of some patients in Germany in 1986, Hamer was struck off and started a strategic pilgrimage to various European countries where he collected new followers and patients and where he was also criminally prosecuted—in France and in Germany with several months of imprisonment—before fleeing in exile to Spain and finally to Norway. Countless television programmes were dedicated to him and although they were mostly critical, they stimulated some complex and dangerous mechanisms of social communication (as we will see better in Chap. 4). This made him the typical representative of alternative therapies for some people: the "independent researcher", "opposed by the powers that be", capable of giving hope "when medicine fails", favourable to a "holistic and natural approach to the disease", "contrary to the use of drugs and chemotherapy" because it is deemed toxic and supported by the economic interests of the pharmaceutical companies. In 2017 alone, in Italy, after having followed the Hamer method, two young women died within a few weeks of one another: in Padua a girl of only 18, and in Rimini a mother of 34 with two children, both with tumoural forms to which the scientifically validated protocols, based on chemotherapy, which both had refused, would have given excellent probabilities of recovery.[8]

As far as Italy is concerned, in the past 40 years, there have been at least three famous cases of therapeutic fraud. In the 1970s, it was the *Bonifacio serum* invented by a veterinary surgeon who imagined treating cancer by giving a distillate of goat's urine to drink (according to the inventor, Liborio Bonifacio, these animals never had cancer); in the 1990s, it was the "alternative anti-tumour therapy", known as the *Di Bella method*, which used a cocktail of drugs based on melatonin, vitamins and hormones (somatostatin) proven to be ineffective by a group of international experts, the results of

---

[8] Rifiuta cure per metodo Hamer, un'altra donna morta a Rimini, Corriere della Sera, 3 Sept. 2016: https://goo.gl/cCNMHd

which were published in the *British Medical Journal*[9]; lastly, between 2007 and 2015 it was the turn of the *Stem cell case* or *Stamina method* (also known as Stamina "therapy" or simply Stamina), in which the journal *Nature*[10] also intervened, in which a non-existent "stem cell-based therapy" was sold at a cost of between euro 30,000 and 50,000, as a treatment for various neurodegenerative diseases. In addition to the risks for the health of the patients, the dramatic aspect of the affair was that the stem cell method was about to be funded by Parliament to the tune of three million euro. This attempt almost succeeded thanks to a skilful media campaign orchestrated by its inventor—a lecturer in psychology and author of a manual of persuasive communication—irresponsibly supported by some television programmes which hid behind the need to "give the news" or "give the patients a voice". The *Stamina method* affair (to which we will return briefly in Chap. 4) ended in 2015 with the plea bargain by its inventor to 1 year and 10 months for criminal conspiracy for the purposes of fraud and with his arrest in 2017 for having repeated the treatment abroad (Capocci and Corbellini 2014; Grignolio and Cattaneo 2014; Cattaneo et al. 2016). Unlike other countries, Italy—where there is a public national health service, extended to all citizens (with a "universalistic" character) and almost free of charge (paid by the taxpayers)—saw in all three cases patients, often demonstrating in the streets, causing a strong emotive impact on the media, making a request to the government to make similar "treatments"—without scientifically proven efficacy—available free of charge in hospitals. This is one of the reasons why in Italy politics, and as a consequence the media, are often involved in these phenomena of charlatanry.

What all the international cases mentioned above have in common is the pernicious media circus that the Internet and TV fuel by acting, more or less involuntarily, as sounding boxes for the fake news and pseudo-science—apart from some praiseworthy TV investigations and blogs which have exposed frauds and false data—trying to exploit populist feelings, increasing clicks and likes for advertising and remunerative purposes, increasing potential TV views or web users to the detriment obviously, of the authority and the reliability of the medical and scientific institutions. These social phenomena linked to pseudo-science, in other words, have anticipated by a few years what other fields of knowledge are today experiencing, from politics to journalism,

---

[9] *Evaluation of an unconventional cancer treatment (the Di Bella multitherapy): results of phase II trials in Italy*. BMJ 1999; 318 (7178): 224–228.

[10] Abbott A. (2013), *Stem-cell ruling riles researchers*, "Nature", 495 (7442), pp. 418–419; Abbott, A. (2013), *Italian stem-cell trial based on flawed data*, "Nature", Jul. 2 2013: https://goo.gl/EUcfE8

or what goes by the name of "post-factual truth" or "post-truth" (as we will see in Chap. 6).

This is the area where vaccines are criticized today in blogs, on the social networks and in the press, even by some recent political movements or representatives—apart from the case of Trump, which will be discussed further, mention must certainly be made of the editorial in *New York Times* regarding the Italian populist movement Cinque Stelle (Five Stars).[11] These are social phenomena based on discrediting experts and suspicion of competences, a phenomenon fuelled by the web which today many define "disintermediation" or the progressive erosion of the authority of the medical and health institutions, based on a misunderstood interpretation of the autonomy of the patient and on a weakness of the doctor's authority (Gray 1999; Kata 2010)—who, however, remains, although with increasing difficulty, one of the social figures in whom Western citizens place the greatest trust. In a comparative international study, the question "Everything considered, do you believe that you can trust a doctor in your country?" was answered as follows: "I very much agree or I agree" by 83% in Switzerland, 79% in Denmark, 78% in the Netherlands, 76% in England and only 58% in the USA (Blendon et al. 2014). In Italy, in particular, before vaccinating their children, 71% of parents rely on their family doctor. The social changes that have come about since the 1980s have inevitably involved a mass preventive treatment like the vaccinal prophylaxis; before then, and for reasons also due to a growing later fertility (as we will see in the next paragraph), few parents would have questioned, as unfortunately is the case today, the authority, the competence and the word of the paediatrician advising them to vaccinate their children.

## An Evolutionary Reason: Late Fertility, Risk, Offspring

Since the dawn of humanity, when our ancestors came down from the trees, taking up an erect position, until 1830, the life expectancy of the human being fluctuated on average between 25 and 35 years—apart from some rare exceptions which concern notable figures, who lived in privileged social contexts and who in general appear in history books. The fact that in the longed-for "bygone times" when "man lived more in contact with nature" on average

---

[11] The Opinion Pages, Editorial, *Populism, Politics and Measles*, "The New York Times", May 2, 2017: https://goo.gl/XpCxvd

he did not reach the age of 40 is something that must always be remembered and which the many adversaries of modernity or technological development should be reminded of. From 1830 onwards, life expectancy gradually increased thanks to the spread of hygiene and health practices—in which, as shown in Chap. 5, vaccinations played a central role (Rappuoli 2014), together with literacy and socio-economic well-being. Today, in the most advanced countries, we have been able to exceed the age of 80, with Italy at the top of the world classification, as in 2015 it could boast of a life expectance of nearly 85 for women and almost 81 for men. In almost two centuries, we have thus tripled the average length of our lives, which even today it gains 3 months every year. Nevertheless, until 1970, families in advanced countries had not changed their average age of fertility, continuing to have children when very young. In other words, for over a century although the average lifespan tripled, parents did not take advantage of the possibility of having children at a later age, still remaining anchored to the times and evolutionary rhythms of our species, but this misalignment between evolution and society did not last long and changed all of a sudden, with effects that are still to be evaluated. The average age of the mother at the birth of her first child, which for a very long time was fairly stable at around 25, progressively increased only from the generations of women born from the second half of the 1950s onwards. Let's have a look at some emblematic cases.

In the USA, between 1991 and 2001, the number of mothers who had their first child between the ages of 35 and 39 increased by 36%, and in the group between 40 and 44 it increased by 70%. The oldest mothers included in this group "are generally better educated and it is more probable that they have more resources, including higher salaries, than mothers who have children when they are younger". On the other hand, from 1990 onwards, the birth rates in the United States decreased amongst all the main ethnic groups: that of the Hispanics, for example, has dropped considerably in the past decades, from 3.0 births per woman in 1990 to 2.4 in 2010, for coloured women from 2.5 to 2.0, and in white women it has dropped, although more slowly from 1.9 to 1.8. In other words, "the fertility rate in the USA is approaching the general European fertility rate, where many countries are fighting very low birth rates (average of 1.6 children per woman)" (Matthews and Hamilton 2009; Matthews et al. 2014; Mather 2012).

In 2015, the total fertility rate of the European Union with 28 states was, to be precise, 1.58 children per woman (the same as in 2014), which is a very low figure, even though it has been comforted by a slight and fluctuating rise in recent years. Amongst the various members, the country that recorded the highest birth rate in 2015 is France, with 1.96 births per woman, the lowest belongs to Portugal with 1.31 children per woman, followed by Poland and Cyprus (1.32), and then by Greece and Spain (1.33). In Europe, furthermore, out of the total of births, the percentage of children born to mothers who are over 40 increased from 1.6% at the end of the 1980s to 3.0% in 2006: if we take the average age of women giving birth in the recent period of time comprised between 2001 and 2015, it has gone from an average of 29.0 to 30.5 years, with England and Germany at the top of the ranking of advanced age mothers in 2009 out of all the 35 countries of the OECD. Another significant piece of data is the fact that many of the women who become pregnant at an advanced age are primipara, especially in the countries characterized by low fertility rates such as Italy and Spain. Amongst the rich countries with a low birth rate, the percentage of births to mothers over 35 grew rapidly from 1980. Exemplary is the case of Austria where the rate of first children born to mothers over 35 was 2% in 1986 whereas in 2014 it had risen to 14%, in the same period the rate of second children went from 5% to 22% (Billari et al. 2011; Beaujouan and Sobotka 2017).[12]

In the United Kingdom as well, the figures show an increase in fertility and in the birth rates of the group of mothers over 35, but if we look at the number of women who have children aged 40, the rate has doubled in the past decade. The statistics show that in 2010, 27,000 children were born to mothers over 40, three times compared to the 9336 in 1989; about one mother out of five is aged 35 or over, and as in the other advanced countries, these more mature mothers tend to be better educated and have greater financial stability. In 2014–2015, the greater percentage increase in the birth rates took place in women over 40 (4.1%), and for women over 40 the rate has more than doubled since 1990.[13]

In Italy today we have reached the average threshold of maternity of 31.5, placing us third in Europe behind Spain and Ireland, where mothers are of an even more advanced age. In 2013/14 in the age-group comprised between 25 and 34, only 36% of women were mothers, also due to postponing maternity: if in 2005–2006, 46.9% of mothers were under 45, in 2013–2014 this percentage was reduced, precisely because the older mothers increased, reaching 42.2%. Italy has another record, that of the least prolific

---

[12] Eurostat. Statistics-explained: Fertility statistics, Mar 2017: https://goo.gl/bjCW8s; OECD Education at a Glance 2013. OECD indicators: https://goo.gl/njQ4G3

[13] UK Office for National Statistics. Statistical bulletin: Conceptions in England and Wales: 2015: https://goo.gl/Zjj9Bc; Older Mum: http://oldermum.co.uk/

European country: 1.4 children per woman on average in 2012 (Istat figures[14]).

In essence, the parents in the more advanced Western countries have increasingly fewer children and increasingly at a later age, which is what statistical studies define a *low and late fertility rate*. It is a clear change for our species, both evolutionary and demographic, which complicates things quite a lot when a parent has to subject their child to a possible medical-health risk.

In recent years, some studies have been devoted to postponed parenthood which can offer some ideas to better contextualize the evolutionary causes that underlie the rejection of vaccinations. The first element that emerges is that with the increase in the age of the parents, the risk of having children with a series of pathologies, including autism, schizophrenia, Down syndrome, various neurocognitive deficiencies, some types of cancer, reduced fertility and longevity also increases (Sandin et al. 2015; Bray et al. 2006; Zhu et al. 2008; Tearne et al. 2015; Heidinger et al. 2016). This data has opened the way for other studies, which show how this type of knowledge has a very significant impact on the perception of risk and, more in general, on the psychological condition of the parents during pregnancy and in the first years of life of their children. During gestation, in particular, the management of feelings linked to uncertainty and the negotiation of the risk about possible diseases of the baby appear, especially in the mother, through an ambivalent relationship with health communication, the motivation and the adhesion to medical recommendations. The various socio-cognitive models used to predict, explain and influence the behaviours of promoting health—the *Health Belief Model*, the *Self-Efficacy Theory*, the theory of *Reasoned Action*, the *Theory of Planned Behaviour*, the *Prospect Theory*, the *Transtheoretical Model*—confirm that the elaborating methods aimed at reducing the perception of risk is one of the commonest strategies adopted by patients (Armitage and Conner 2000; Munro et al. 2007; Sutton 2008). Exposed to the risk of diseases of their babies and the uncertainty of the result of the birth, as well as of the reduced probability of having other reproductive chances, advanced age parents tend to reduce anxiety-inducing situations in communications with healthcare operators, avoiding the negative information on the age-related risks and focusing rather on a healthy lifestyle linked to diet, physical activity and mental and physical well-being (Bayrampour et al. 2012). Another significant

---

[14] ISTAT. Come cambia la vita delle donne 2004–2014, http://tinyurl.com/jkw546v. Avere figli in Italia negli anni 2000. Approfondimenti dalle indagini campionarie sulle nascite e sulle madri, http://tinyurl.com/h3tawce

consequence of this delicate anxiety-inducing condition is that mothers in particular rely on self-taught health information—through the Internet, articles in the press and various informative material. However, in the medium term, this approach is often useless and a cause of anguish, both due to the quantity of data available and its contradictory nature. Doctors and healthcare operators find this attitude very difficult to control because, unlike the parents, who tend to base their information on a subjective evaluation of the risk based on personal experience or individual real stories, often from their entourage of family or friends—a bias which, as we will see in the conclusions, will be used to convince the parents contrary to vaccinations—they have knowledge based on epidemiological data which orients them towards an objective assessment of the risk (Carolan and Nelson 2007; Carolan 2009; Lampinen et al. 2009).

This condition of emotive fragility increases with the advanced (34–38) and very advanced age (39 and over) when they become parents of a first child, in relation to the post-birth phase and the first 3 years of the child's life. With respect to younger parents, these two groups of mature parents show greater mental problems such as depressive syndrome, anxiety linked to uncertainty, sleeping problems, prolonged stress and tiredness (Nilsen et al. 2012, 2013; Aasheim et al. 2012, 2014). This data is also confirmed by the analyses which test the degree of existential satisfaction in the absence of maternity and during it, at an increasing age: it appears clear that existential malaise of the parents increases gradually from 28 to 40–42 (Blanchflower and Oswald 2008) and reaches a maximum when the child is about three, with the most dissatisfied parent age group between the ages of 36 and 40; moreover, these data contradict the theory according to which there is a compensation between the greater socioeconomic solidity of adult parents and the health and psychological risks to which they are exposed (Aasheim et al. 2014).

These studies suggest different things. In the first place, that autism and other neurocognitive disabilities that the anti-vaccination movements relate mistakenly to the use of the MMR vaccine, in actual fact increase with the gradual advance of the average age of parenthood, which includes the majority of the parents who oppose vaccinations for fears linked to their neurotoxic effects. In the second place, these data suggest that when these parents go to the paediatrician for the vaccinations in the first 3 years of life of their child, they are in a psychological condition of discomfort, due both to the uncertainty for the possible congenital diseases of their child (accentuated by unreliable and contradictory online information) and to the parental and existential stress due to their advanced age. The latter often coincides with reaching a social status and the formation of a more structured identity by the parents and these characteristics probably favour behaviour, unimaginable until a few decades ago, going against the authority and the advice of the doctor or paediatrician: a parent of 40 is certainly more likely, compared to a 20-year-old parent, to ignore the invitation of the paediatrician to vaccinate their child. This socio-cognitive context, in addition to the absence of siblings and the scarce possibility of leaving further descendants, creates a combined effect of a maximum perception of the risk towards the offspring and therefore a maximum capacity to assess possible health choices in the wrong way.

Therefore, having a lot of information on the risk does not lead individuals to make correct health decisions (Gigerenzer 2015; Gigerenzer and Gray 2013) as, due to the evolution of our brain, in contexts of uncertainty, it makes suboptimal and irrational decisions, as shown by the model of "bounded rationality" of Kahneman (2012). In the prospect theory, perhaps the most predictive theory of decision-making choices of recent years, Kahneman shows that human choices are characterized by an aversion to risk—with the figures at stake being equal, the perception of a possible economic loss always dominates that of a possible win, as well as of an over-estimation of the importance of improbable events. In other words, ancestral behaviour to defend their offspring is triggered in the mind of parents but it turns out to be irrational and counter-productive. For parents in a generalized situation of stress, even if there is only the slightest possibility of jeopardizing the life of their only descendant, they overestimate the remote possibility of adverse events and avoidance of risk. It is, however, a suboptimal estimation or, better, a very bad one.

In order to protect children, nothing is safer than a life insurance like vaccinations, which immunize them against potentially fatal infections. Not doing so is like sending a child out on a motorbike without a helmet or in a dangerous car, indeed it is a far worse risk as, to give only two examples, in 2014 in Italy there were 55.6 fatalities (and more than 4000 casualties) in road accidents every million inhabitants, whilst in 2013 in the USA, there were 106 deaths out of a million, against one person out of a million who shows a severe adverse reaction, but not death, towards a vaccination.[15]

---

[15] ISTAT. Incidenti stradali, Anno 2014, http://tinyurl.com/glsden2; WHO. *Violence and Injury Prevention. Global status report on road safety 2015.* USA p. 248: https://goo.gl/RF8trm

# 2

# A Brief History of Anti-vaccination Movements

## The Anti-vaccination Movements in the Eighteenth and Nineteenth Centuries: Obligation and Objection

The story of the anti-vaccination movements, which have opposed vaccinations for health, religious and political reasons, is a story that is as old as the very practice of inoculating smallpox (Moulin 1996). In this long story, however, there has not been a single case where the movements have raised fears that the scientific community has deemed as having any grounds. However, they have at times reached results both in a legal context, obtaining in some cases exemption from compulsory vaccinations, and in the context of the pharmaceutical production. In one case, they succeeded having a preservative, unjustly deemed toxic, eliminated. Similar results, as will be seen, represent an apparent victory because they have not given any effective advantage to the anti-vaccination movements and, most importantly, at times they have even decreased herd immunity by causing new outbreaks of epidemics.

It was from the early eighteenth century that a preventive health practice spread in Europe against the epidemics of smallpox known as *variolation*, i.e. the practice of immunizing healthy people infecting them (through a superficial scarification on the arm) with pus from vesicles from people affected by reduced forms of smallpox, according to the principle that once the disease has been contracted lifelong immunity to it is acquired (for the history of vaccination, see Chap. 5). Smallpox, as we will see, is a virus which since

© Springer International Publishing AG, part of Springer Nature 2018
A. Grignolio, *Vaccines: Are they Worth a Shot?*, https://doi.org/10.1007/978-3-319-68106-1_2

10,000 BC has terrified thousands of generations with its cyclical outbreaks of epidemics. Its mortality rate is 30–355; it disfigures survivors' faces and in the eighteenth century alone caused the death of 75 million people (about 10% of the world population of the time). Even though England was the first European country to import the health prophylaxis of variolation from the Orient, it was in one of its colonies that it became most firmly established and, consequently, encountered the first fierce disagreements.

On 22 April 1721, the Seahorse, a vessel coming from the Caribbean, docked in the port of Boston, one of the main cities of New England, carrying with her spices, various commodities and, as was learnt later, a crew suffering from smallpox. New England had already several epidemics: in 1677, in the 2 years 1689/90 and in 1702, and Boston had already observed since 1648 the cautionary procedure of waiting for 40 days, the so-called quarantine, before allowing vessels at risk to dock. Yet, in that spring of 1721 nothing seemed able to stem the epidemic, which spread very quickly in the city. Under the guidance of the Reverend Cotton Mather, trained at Harvard and a convinced advocate of variolation—thanks also to the stories of his coloured butler, Onesimus, who had undergone variolation in his native Africa (Herbert 1975)—and the city's doctor Zabdiel Boylston, the Boston area was subjected to a systematic programme of inoculation which encountered some areas of resistance both in the population and in the medical community. On the days of the greatest spread of the epidemic, a radical fringe of the groups contrary to variolation even made an attempt on the life of the reverend, throwing a bomb into his apartment with a threatening message.

Without losing heart, Mather and Boylston decided that the best response would have come from the transparency of scientific data—although, to tell the truth, Mather seems to have forgotten about this method 20 years later in relation to the women accused of witchcraft in the Salem trial. They were the first in the world to use a comparative strategic approach, comparing the mortality rate caused by the infection of smallpox with that caused by variolation. Their conclusions were unequivocal: during the great epidemic of 1721, about half of the 12,000 citizens of Boston contracted smallpox; 14% of them had died when infected by the natural form, while only 2% of those infected by variolation died. Despite this enormous success, Mather's method did not succeed in immediately convincing the authorities of the New World. We can perhaps think of the best known historical case. In 1776, the army of General George Washington, weakened by an epidemic of smallpox, failed to wrench Quebec from the British army, stronger because it was immune due to the compulsory variolation of the soldiers. Having learned the lesson, the next year, Washington variolated his army, which changed not only the fate of his soldiers, but his decision played a crucial role in the process which led to the independence and the creation of the United States. It also helped him indirectly take up the position of the first President of the new country (Aronson and Newman 2002; Riedel 2005).

The first real anti-vaccination groups, however, were formed only in the early nineteenth century with the spread of vaccination. This practice had been introduced in England thanks to the British doctor Edward Jenner (1749–1823). He proved, with a note sent to the Royal Society in 1798, the greater safety and efficacy of immunization through infection with the small-pox vaccine (a practice called vaccination) instead of, as was then in vogue, using vesicles of human smallpox. The first caricature by the best known cartoonist of the period, James Gillray, was of 1803, in which Jenner is ridiculed while he vaccinates several terrified people, with small cows sprouting from their various orifices and the points of inoculation. On the other hand, the English authorities, evidently insensitive to popular fears, immediately understood the importance of the discovery and launched a mass vaccinal prophylaxis, regulating it in time with various legislative measures. The first was the *Vaccination Act* of 1840, which made vaccinations free for the poor and prohibited the previous practice of variolation (then defined *inoculation*). However, it was not until 1853 that vaccination became compulsory by law for children from three months of age, and a fine was introduced for objectors. In 1867, the compulsory age was raised to 14, and fairly harsh provisions were introduced, such as a trial with a brief procedure and heavy fines for parents who were unable to certify the vaccination of their children, as well as prison for those who produced or spread vaccine serums that were not regulatory. These measures represented a significant stage of interference by the state into civil liberties in the name of public health and from the start were opposed.

Following the 1853 law, there were already violent clashes with the police in some British towns such as Ipswich, Henley and Mitford. These first move-ments did not accept the attempt by the public institutions to protect citizens from the continuous outbreaks of smallpox and perceived the legislative actions as damaging to individual liberty. The opponents included a fair number of parents who refused that their children be inoculated with infected pus from strangers. Others, including a part of the clergy, opposed in the name of the promiscuity, considered "unchristian", between animal and human blood (Durbach 2000). Others put forward their own arguments in favour of a general mistrust in medicine. There was even a minority of doctors who defined vaccination a dubious practice based on a superseded method—i.e. deemed too similar to the principle according to which "like cures like" (*similia similibus curantur*), typical of prescientific medicine and advocated by

Paracelsus (1493–1541), who, together with Samuel Hahnemann (1755–1843), is today considered the father of homeopathy (Kayne 2006; Bellavite et al. 2005). All this was despite the fact that the rate of mortality of smallpox had reached between 20 and 30% of the people affected by the natural infection, compared to only 2% of variolated people. This mortality rate, subsequently understood, was also due to the poor hygienic practices of inoculation and the transmission of other venereal infections through the exchange of infected blood (Huth 2006; Porter and Porter 1988).

Following the 1867 law, which harshened the compulsory nature of vaccinations, the first associations of anti-vaccinationists were formed, such as the Anti-Compulsory Vaccination League, which was organized at national level and promoted the publication of various magazines of vulgarization. The protests continued, even though in 1871, a new wave of smallpox in England had caused over 20,000 victims. In 1885, the city of Leicester witnessed an important protest march, in which 80,000 people accompanied a mother and 2 men who had refused to vaccinate their children to the local police station. Similar events made the institutions designate the Royal Commission on Vaccination. After 7 years of intense work in which the various parties in dispute were scrupulously listened to—making the data of the scientific community equivalent to the beliefs and opinions of non-experts, a recurring and lasting political strategy of consent as we will see—in 1896 the Commission certified the efficacy and the safety of the vaccination, but suggested the suspension of the penalties for objectors. This was followed by the *Vaccination Act* of 1898, which eliminated to all effects the penalties and introduced the clause of "conscientious objection" for parents who refused vaccination. From then on, parents could obtain a certificate of exemption (Wolfe and Sharp 2002). In actual fact, the British authorities were rather skilful in holding together the freedoms requested by the citizens and the need for a sufficient vaccinal coverage, forcing the conscientious objectors to face a series of fairly elaborate bureaucratic procedures. Before obtaining the certificate of exemption, the anti-vaccination parents had to prove that their conviction as conscientious objectors was authentic before two magistrates and one stipendiary who often declared they were not satisfied and reiterated the issue of the certificate at their pleasure—which had to come about, on pain of annulation, within 4 months of the birth of the child. Following numerous appeals, in 1907, there was another *Vaccination Act*. On the one hand, it established the obligation of the magistrates to sign the requests of the reluctant parents; on the other it imposed on the latter a complicated bureaucratic procedure, in the course of which they had to, inter alia, show in writing the responsibility of refusing a safe and consolidated practice which exposed their children to the risk of fatal diseases. In this way, the British institutions succeeded in keeping under control the number of people exempt from vaccinal coverage, which in 1906 did not exceed 1% of the population.

Similar movements sprung up in different parts of Europe, but not all the institutions were as skilful as the British. In mid-nineteenth century Stockholm, most of the population started to refuse the vaccination, and in 1872, they dropped to a minimum level to cover only 40% of the city's population—a rate which, as mentioned, annuls the precious herd immunity—while keeping a rate of 90% in the rest of rural Sweden. The medical and health authorities of the city, directed by Dr. C. A. Grähs, launched repeated appeals to the population on the possible repeated risks, but systematically they went unheard. In 1874, the outbreak of a new wave of epidemics began to sow death again and rekindled the perception of the risk in the city's population, who began to be vaccinated again: the anti-vaccination movements stopped and with them the return of future epidemics of smallpox to Sweden (Nelson and Rogers 1992). In the United States as well, after a first phase of enthusiasm which led to a sharp drop in the epidemics of smallpox, various groups of people scattered throughout the country came together around anti-vaccination feelings. Starting from 1870, the insufficient group immunity rekindled the infectious foci and the US health institutions attempted to pass new laws in favour of vaccination which found marginal, but highly active, groups of resistance. The visit to New York by William Tebb, the best known anti-vaccination activist of the time, persuaded the first groups to set up the Anti-Vaccination Society of America in 1879, followed, 3 years later, by the New England Anti-Compulsory Vaccination League and, in 1885, by the Anti-Vaccination League of New York City. Through the production of booklets, the organization of legal battles in the courts, public protests and, not infrequently, clashes with the police (as in Milwaukee, or in the Canadian city of Montreal), some groups were able to obtain the abrogation of compulsory vaccination in a number of states, including California (Kaufman 1967). In this context, the case of Henning Jacobson was exemplary: in 1902, following vaccinations becoming compulsory to meet an epidemic of smallpox in Massachusetts, he refused vaccination, appealing to the right to treat himself according to his personal convictions. The city authorities of Cambridge started criminal proceedings against him, who opposed them and lost, taking his legal battle to the Supreme Court. In 1905, it did not uphold his reasons, establishing the right of the State to issue compulsory laws when there are diseases that endanger the safety of society—it was a historic decision, as it was the first case in which the highest legislative body of the United States granted full powers to the federal states on regulating public health (Albert et al. 2001; Gostin 2005).

# The Anti-vaccination Movements in the Twentieth Century: The Media and Politics

Towards the end of the nineteenth century, the attention of the anti-vaccination movements moved from legal questions to those linked to the dangerousness of vaccinations and to conspiracy theories, up to the rejection of traditional medicine in the name of an approach that was "naturalist", "environmentalist", "holistic" or "alternative". An interesting comparative study has shown how these beliefs have remained virtually unchanged over 200 years of history, proving once again how some fears are deeply rooted, presumably at neurophysiological level, and what the classic mechanisms of reaction of the perceived risk are. All these beliefs were already shown in the "National Anti-Compulsory Vaccination Reporter" (Cheltenham, England) in 1878, which accused the vaccination against smallpox of causing serious illnesses (diphtheria and fatal cutaneous septicaemia such as erysipelas, known as St Anthony's fire), of being ineffective, of being replaceable by naturist lifestyles and practices that were more effective in immunizing the organism, of using substances deemed poisonous (phenic acid) in the inoculation procedures, of fuelling the despotic and paternalistic attitude of the health institutions with the intention of dominating the population and, lastly, of offering an immunity cover limited in time, with the obligation of repeated and dangerous booster injections (Wolfe and Sharp 2002). These criticisms remained constant in the first decades of the twentieth century, even though they underwent a setback thanks to the vertiginous development of vaccinations which between 1930 and 1960 eradicated all the main infectious diseases that had afflicted the history of humanity. Except for intermediate and marginal cases, it was not until the 1970s that there was a return of the anti-vaccination movements. If, on the one hand, they reproposed the same classic criticisms as always, on the other hand they acquired in this period of time effective communication strategies proving to be more capable than their adversaries (doctors and scientific institutions) in using the media and other propaganda instruments to spread their ideas. The most traumatic event that concerns the vaccination movements in the second half of the twentieth century is without any doubt the Wakefield fraud against the MMR vaccine, which will be discussed in greater detail later (in Chap. 4), but few people remember that in the 1970s there was a violent campaign of disinformation against another vaccination, that against diphtheria, tetanus and whooping cough (known as DTP). It was perhaps the first media campaign against vaccinations promoted at worldwide level.

Towards the end of the 1960s, the vaccination for whooping cough had been able to effectively contain the spread of this infection in the West—according to the WHO in 2003 it still affected 17.6 million individuals, killing almost 3,00,000 (mostly children). The health authorities were aware that the vaccination was imperfect and with a low rate of efficacy compared to the others, so they established the doses according to specific circumstances linked to the age and health conditions of the population. This was a reason that the anti-vaccinationists deemed sufficient to fuel doubts and movements against its spread. The spark that triggered off collective fear broke out in 1974 with the circulation of a report by the Great Ormond Street Hospital in London. According to this report, neurological complications were hypothesized in 36 children following the invocation of the vaccination against pertussis. Television documentaries, newspaper articles and an "association of parents of children damaged by vaccinations" fuelled the controversy, causing a sudden drop in the rates of vaccination. An inquiry committee and an independent committee of experts were set up who confirmed that the vaccination was safe. These reassurances by scientific committees left British citizens in a state of uncertainty, instigated by some isolated cases of doctors doubtful about the vaccinations and in particular by one, Gordon Stewart, who put himself at the head of the opponents leading the anti-vaccination movement. A costly national programme for infantile encephalopathy became necessary, which analysed all children aged between 24 and 36 months in the hospitals of the United Kingdom for neurological diseases, in order to establish through statistical evidence that the vaccinations were not responsible and annul the many lawsuits seeking compensation. The activity of disinformation carried out by the anti-vaccination movements in the United Kingdom was such that the cover for pertussis, which in the 1960s had reached 81% of the population, in the mid-1970s plummeted to 31%. As on other occasions in the past, the absence of herd immunity allowed the bacteria of pertussis (*Bordetella pertussis*) to start spreading again in the British population: further evidence that the bacteria are almost never defeated by vaccination but only kept at bay. Unfortunately, the most foreseeable conclusion came about; following the events of the Great Ormond Hospital an epidemic of whooping cough broke out in the United Kingdom and the medical and health institutions and the citizens took remedial action with mass vaccination, which soon reached 93% of the population. That was the last time that a focus of pertussis affected England, until the recent cases of 2012 which will be discussed later (Miller and Ross 1978; Baker 2003).

News of these events reached and spread to Asia, Australia and the United States where, in 1982, a documentary against the MMR vaccination was produced and in 1991 a book was published on its potential risks for health. Associations of parents and pressure groups against vaccinations were also immediately created in the United States but, unlike the British ones, the US scientific and health institutions responded energetically and immediately. There were television programmes that chased audiences by riding on the fears of the population, a number of lawsuits were started against the pharmaceutical companies (some of which decided, as we will see, to suspend the production of the incriminated vaccine for economic reasons) and there was even a rise in the price of the vaccines. Nevertheless, the drop in vaccinations against diphtheria, tetanus and pertussis was more contained than in Great Britain (Gangarosa 1998).

Two decades later, in 1998, England was again the scene of a new wave of fears against vaccinations, started by the Wakefield affair (see Chap. 4), but immediately afterwards it was the United States that had to face a major anti-vaccination movement, the last known today at worldwide level. Towards the end of the 1990s, doubts began to rise on the harmfulness of an excipient to preserve the vaccine: thimerosal or thiomersal. It was suspected of containing a neurotoxic component like mercury. Before the discovery of antiseptic molecules, mercury and its derivatives were often used in the biomedical field for their well-known bactericide and fungicide properties and from 1930 onwards, the companies manufacturing vaccines started to use thiomersal to sterilize the multi-use packaging of the vaccines. The vials came into contact with several syringes (also multi-use) and this had originated severe episodes of infection, in 1916 in the United States and in 1928 in Australia. The substance contained in thiomersal accused by the American anti-vaccinationists in the 1990s was ethylmercury, completely harmless and rapidly eliminated by the organism, which was confused with methylmercury, a molecule that is neurotoxic by accumulation, but which has nothing to do with vaccines. The *m* that distinguishes ethylmercury from methylmercury is essential, because in the language of chemistry it refers to two different molecules (one atom of carbon and two of hydrogen more or less). The three atoms have a similar difference, for example, in distinguishing methanol, a powerful poison—which in the mid-1980s was at the centre of the Italian methanol-tainted wine scandal which caused about 20 victims (Suro 1986)—from ethanol, the harmless form of alcohol typically present in wine (Rappuoli and Vozza 2009, p. 44). When the bactericide thiomersal, based on ethylmercury, was included in vaccines, the Food and Drug Administration (FDA), the US regulating body for drugs, decided to do so with, as always, all the necessary caution. It used low doses that would have been harmless even for the toxic methylmercury—at tiny doses, even poisons are tolerated—and tested them on laboratory animals and on their foetuses, which are notoriously more sensitive, without the slightest side effect being ascertained.[1] Not even today, after years and millions of individuals who have been vaccinated, are there any contraindications or adverse effects worthy of note (Andrews et al. 2004).

Two historical precedents also completely absolved thiomersal: in the state of Indiana in 1929, it was tested to treat an epidemic of meningitis with doses equal to 10,000 times that contained in the vaccines, without showing signs of toxicity (Baker 2008); and towards the end of the 1980s the effect of the toxic methylmercury, which was absorbed in high doses by the population, was also analysed, without this showing any neurological damage. This case is part of a vast epidemiological study—a medical discipline that uses extensive statistical data to understand the distribution and frequency of diseases in the population, both for preventive purposes and to reconstruct a posteriori causes or correlations that are not evident—conducted in the mid-1980s. In this case, the high doses of methylmercury present in the fish eaten by mothers on some islands of the Seychelles were analysed to assess the possible neurological damage on their foetuses. The results, published in "The Lancet", one of the most authoritative scientific journals in the world, confirmed that the children, although raised on fish rich in methylmercury, in their subsequent development did not show any difference or cognitive disease compared to the control group represented by children in the United States who ate food free of mercury (Myers et al. 2003).

Going back to the harmless ethylmercury, the American anti-vaccination activists loudly demanded its removal for precautionary purposes according to a poorly understood "principle of precaution", one of the rhetorical instruments most used by those who oppose vaccines and, more in general, by those with an attitude of mistrust towards science (see Chap. 3). Science had already taken the precautions, as we have just seen, about 70 years earlier with thiomersal; yet the strategy of involving completely inexpert people but skilful in communicating, such as actors and celebrities, defeated the overwhelming evidence offered by the scientific method. The Green Our Vaccines movement, headed by the well-known actor Jim Carrey and by the playmate Jenny McCarthy, was founded, with a campaign centred on the idea of "removing the toxins" from vaccines, that were believed capable of causing autism. The campaign had a fair success in the media and other associations (Generation rescue) and associations of parents with children suffering from autism (Talk About curing Autism) joined it. To avoid the drop in coverage, in 1999, some

---

[1] Centers for Disease Control and Prevention (CDC), Understanding Thimerosal, Mercury, and Vaccine Safety, http://tinyurl.com/n8ejv5g

U.S. health institutions and pharmaceutical companies decided to eliminate, or at least decrease, the thiomersal from many vaccines. It was a sensible decision, but which gave the idea that against irrational social pressure the institutions for collective public health could give in, opening up the way to further unjustified accusations, as in fact happened.

After the drastic reduction of thiomersal in the vaccines, however, there was no drop at all in the number of cases of autism: this not only exonerated the molecule which was the object of prejudicial attacks, but proves, once again, how the confrontation with the anti-vaccination activists must be based not on empirical data but rather on a narrative and emotional dimension which takes into account the cognitive biases (distortions of the ability of judgement) suggested by neuroscience (as will be shown in Chap. 6).

The case of ethylmercury is not an isolated one, as in recent years the anti-vaccine movements have been mounting accusations against other components. As will be discussed in the next paragraph, harmless molecules were branded as toxic, such as squalene, a biological component that stimulates the immune response and is also produced naturally by humans, and formaldehyde, a substance that is used toinactivate viruses and toxins in sone specific vaccines. Supposed "heavy metals" present in the vials were also accused. Although part of the accusations still believe that these "toxic components" cause the onset of autism or various other neurological diseases, in the past few years the cancer interpretation has been gaining ground, i.e. the idea that the toxicity of these additives in vaccines causes cancer. The so-called vaccine overload is also accused of the same thing, believed to cause the onset of tumours through weakening the immune system.

In the United States, alongside actors (Robert De Niro, Charlie Sheen, Kirstie Alley), television presenters (Bill Maher) and various celebrities (Robert F. Kennedy Jr.), there is also a small group of politicians who criticize vaccines in various ways, such as the former Secretary of State John Kerry, the tycoon and current President of the United States, Donald Trump,[2] the former Democratic senators Joe Lieberman and Chris Dodd and the Republican

---

[2] On Twitter, there are at least four messages by Donald Trump which are critical of vaccinations, two of which even establish the link—the result, as we will see of a well-known scientific fraud which over 100 experiments had proven to be completely unfounded—between autism and vaccines, for example the tweet of 28 March 2014: "Healthy young child goes to doctor, gets pumped with massive shot of many vaccines, doesn't feel good and changes—AUTISM. Many such cases!". On the same subject, see also the articles by Lena H. Sun, "Trump energizes the anti-vaccine movement in Texas", *The Washington Post*, Feb 20, 2017; by Sarah Kaplan, "The truth about vaccines, autism and Robert F. Kennedy Jr.'s conspiracy theory", *The Washington Post*, January 10 2017; and by Michael D. Shear, Maggie Haberman and Pam Belluck, "Anti-Vaccine Activist Says Trump Wants Him to Lead Panel on Immunization Safety". *The New York Times*, Jan 10, 2017.

Congresswoman Michele Bachmann (Ołpiński 2012). As in the rest of the Western world, American actors are also inclined to naturism and alternative treatments to medicine—John Travolta and Tom Cruise, for example, have been followers of Scientology, a religious organization critical of psychiatry and a supporter of "alternative" approaches to psychiatric diseases, including autism (Chesworth 2005; Shermer 2011; Kent and Manca 2013)[3] and some go as far as to spread critical theories against vaccines (Robert De Niro, Charlie Sheen, Kirstie Alley, Jim Carrey, Jenny McCarthy). Sometimes, it is because they have been personally affected by family dramas and pathologies which persuade them to abandon scientifically proven treatment and protocols. The most recent and famous case is that of the actor Robert De Niro who, in 2016, as the co-founder of the Tribeca Film Festival in New York, after having proposed including in the festival programme a documentary on the rehabilitation of Andrew Wakefield and his false relationship between vaccines and autism, decided to withdraw it following the heated controversy and the intervention of various scientific institutions (Lee 2016; Cha 2016).

In Italy as well, where recently a political movement has become established which expresses doubts on vaccinations, the 5 Star Movement,[4] opposition to vaccines, is gaining ground and the monitoring centres notice a drop in coverage, especially for the MMR vaccine. At least three critical areas, such as that between Cesena and Rimini, in central Italy, one in the north around the city of Bolzano and in the south in some parts of Sicily[5] are concerned. For about 10 years, various groups of anti-vaccinationists have been launching on the Internet a series of false accusations against vaccines which in the end have reached, and evidently convinced, politicians of various leanings. Unfortunately, we will hear about this recent return of anti-intellectualism, in which the Internet facilitates non-scientific and conspiracy theories being transmitted into the heart of the political institutions, very often in the coming years (Broadbent 2017; Kuntz 2017; McDevitt et al. 2017; Berezow 2017; Rose et al. 2016; Sternhell 2010).

---

[3] Yahr, E., "How Scientology controls John Travolta and Tom Cruise, according to 'Going Clear'", *The Washington Post*, March 30, 2015: https://goo.gl/KjasVU

[4] See, for example, the editorial of *The New York Times* of May 2 2017, "Populism, Politics and Measles" which discusses the fact that : "Beppe Grillo, the leader of the populist Five Star Movement in Italy, has campaigned actively on an anti-vaccination platform".

[5] Epicentro. Il portale dell'epidemiologia per la sanità pubblica, edited by the Centro Nazionale di Epidemiologia, Sorveglianza e Promozione della Salute. Coperture vaccinali nell'infanzia 2009. Regione Emilia-Romagna—Assessorato Politiche per la Salute, pp. VIII, XI: http://tinyurl.com/hu6tw7s; Regione Emilia-Romagna. Assessorato Politiche per la Salute, Coperture vaccinali nell'infanzia e nell'adolescenza Anno 2014, http://www.epicentro.iss.it/

Raising general doubts as, for example, some groups of anti-vaccinationists have done in the past, accusing multiple vaccinations of weakening the immune system of soldiers, or as more recently Donald Trump and Robert F. Kennedy Jr. have done, accusing them of creating autism in children, possibly hoping with political rhetoric in a future programme of checking the vaccination patterns, is more effective from the media's point of view than referring to empirical data. Yet, studies that deny the side effects of multiple vaccinations, in the short and long term, are already widely available in the most accredited literature (Gregson and Edelman 2003; Pittman et al. 2004; Broderick et al. 2015). The subject clearly has a political force and has become so common, especially amongst parents at grips with paediatric vaccinations such as the trivalent or hexavalent vaccinations that it is specifically treated on the sites of the most important international institutions for public health and the control of the vaccinal prophylaxis (Miller et al. 2003; Hilton et al. 2006). In actual fact, understanding that multiple vaccination is a false problem is fairly simple, and it is an explanation that applies both to soldiers as well as to children. In a single school year, children in the first 5 years of their life receive an immune stimulation tens of times greater than those of the vaccines, thanks to the natural cyclical infections which affect classrooms an average of 4–6 times a year. The human immune system is very strong and, although in small children it is still developing, we have to consider that every millilitre of their blood contains ten million cells (lymphocyte b) which are responsible for the antibody response, estimated sufficient to cope with something like 10,000 vaccines at a time (Offit et al. 2002). It has also been proven that combining all the vaccines in a single inoculation, as well as reducing stress for the children and being a more economical solution for families (WHO 2009), by no means reduces their efficacy. Above all, however, to frame the false problem, one technical element of absolute significance has to be made known: if it is true that the number of vaccines required has increased over the years, it is equally true that the number of molecules (antigens) capable of activating an immunological response has also dropped sharply. To give one example, consider that in 1960 there were no fewer than 3200 antigens (immunostimulant molecules) in the four vaccines that protected from the same number of infectious diseases, whereas by 2012, 60 components have been obtained that are capable of protecting us against eleven diseases: meningococcus B alone, the commonest of the five types of bacteria that cause meningitis in Europe, contains about 90 immunogenetic proteins.

In theory anyone who raises doubts, especially in the institutions, should be acquainted with the specific literature and indicate whether there are data that they believe unreliable, instead of continuing to reiterate old fears that have now been solved. Unfortunately, in reality, this is not how the relationship between science, society and politics works, and often storytelling, based on conspiracy theories, which accuses the pharmaceutical companies of acting against public health is more successful than the message according to which they, monitored and stimulated by the public and regulatory institutions, compete to increase the well-being and average life expectancy of citizens—a fact which appears obvious from any investigations without preconceptions and based on data (see Chap. 5). As has been seen in this brief overview of history, over the past three centuries not a single fear raised by the anti-vaccinationists has been confirmed by scientific data. A similar conclusion, when all is said and done, also applies to the legal context focused on the exemption of obligatoriness.

There are countries that recommend vaccinations, those that encourage them and others that consider them compulsory, mainly as certification required for school enrolment. The world panorama on the compulsory nature of paediatric vaccinations is extremely heterogeneous and in all the Western countries (and in non-Western ones characterized by a medium socio-economic development), sufficient coverage is achieved to obtain herd immunity independently of the compulsory nature. Here are, in brief, the different choices of the different countries.

In Great Britain, compulsory vaccination, for which the way was led by the anti-vaccination movements, was reached in 1948. Although without obligation, British citizens diligently followed the health authorities, with some significant exceptions which caused severe waves of epidemics: in 1950 there was a last outbreak of smallpox in Glasgow, and at the end of the 1970s, as we have seen, an epidemic of whooping cough; while in very recent years there was an epidemic of whooping cough in 2012 (with almost 10,000 cases and the death of 14 babies under 3 months[6]), 6 in 2013 and 3 in 2014,[7] as well as an epidemic of measles between 2012 and 2013, attributable to the Wakefield fraud with 3800 cases (10,271 in Europe in 2013 alone).

In 2017, Germany introduced a law to fine (up to 2500 €) parents who do not report to the authorities their refusal to vaccinate their children when enrolling them at the nursery (Escritt 2017).

In North America, the individual states, as well as the various provinces of Canada, decide autonomously: out of the 50 states, a fair number (28) admit exemption for medical, religious and philosophical reasons, a smaller number (19) also accept philosophical reasons (personal convictions) except Mississippi, West Virginia and (recently) California, which only allow exemption for

---

[6] Oxford Vaccine group, Vaccine Knowledge Project, Pertussis (whooping cough), http://tinyurl.com/pjfraj3

[7] Public Health England, Research and analysis, "HPR", volume 9, issue 30, news (28 August), Laboratory Confirmed Pertussis in England, Data to End-June 2015, http://tinyurl.com/l4soqef

medical reasons (compromise of the immune system or severe illnesses) (Pierik 2017). In particular, out of the 48 contiguous states (excluding Alaska and Hawaii) 25 require a simple declaration, 15 require from parents a document with a legalized signature in which they declare that they are aware of putting their child in a situation of risk and 9 impose a highly structured procedure. It is a composite situation in which, however, it has been proven—as English history of the late nineteenth century had already suggested—that the more the bureaucratic procedure is structured, informative and puts parents before their responsibilities, the lower the percentage of objectors and therefore the number of epidemics that break out (Rota et al. 2001; Bradford and Mandich 2015). The recent case of California is emblematic. In June 2015, the governor of California, Jerry Brown, tightened the State rules for exemption from vaccination (Senate Bill 277) because of the worrying outbreak of an epidemic of measles. Between 17 and 20 December 2014, at Disneyland in Anaheim, California, there were several cases of measles that started to spread with a worrying speed, reaching, in the following weeks, almost 150 cases in different US states, expanding to Canada and Mexico (Phadke et al. 2016). This is an evident demonstration of how, in the face of the onset of infection, the American population is below the threshold of herd immunity. Some studies connect this effect to the campaigns of "growing anti-vaccination movements and the prevalence of hesitant parents" towards vaccinations (Majumder et al. 2015; Nagourney 2015). The drop in cover is a great risk for all citizens, but it is a real disaster for the most fragile part of the population, as the two stories below remind us.

In 2015, in Port Angeles, in the state of Washington, Catherina Montantes was working as a dental hygienist in a medical surgery to pay for her criminology studies: her dream, never fulfilled, was to become a border police officer. She was 28 and a few months earlier she had been diagnosed with an inflammatory disease (dermatomyositis) which she had to treat with immunosuppressant drugs that lowered her immune defence capacities. At the end of January, during a hospital examination, she was one of the three dozen people infected by a patient with measles, a 52-year-old man who was the first case of measles in 20 years in the area of Clallam County and who was able to infect 149 people in a few days. Bad luck meant that Catherina did not develop the classic symptoms of measles and the virus replicated almost asymptomatically for 6 weeks until she was admitted to hospital on 19 March and she died on 8 April due to pneumonia caused by measles, as confirmed by the autopsy and the blood tests (Burioni 2016).[8] For the reintroduction of compulsory

---

[8] Aleccia, J., *'Go-getter' with hopes of a new career: the Port Angeles woman felled by the measles*, The Seattle Times, April 21, 2016 (https://goo.gl/oSqw3y).

vaccination, the media event triggered off by the story of Rhett Krawitt was significant. Rhett was a Californian child aged 6 whose leukaemia in remission after effective chemotherapy (but with a momentarily compromised immune system) left him vulnerable to infectious diseases and he could not have an anti-measles vaccination. His father appealed to the competent authorities, stating that, like all immune-depressed people, the life of his son was guaranteed by the immunity of the community and that it was seriously endangered by some unvaccinated pupils at Rhett's school, the coverage rate of which was lower than the other schools in the Bay Area of San Francisco (Lewinjan 2015). As soon as the law made vaccinations compulsory again, the Californian anti-vaccination movements called a referendum to try and abolish it, but without reaching a sufficient number of signatures (McGreevy 2015). In June 2015, the American Medical Association approved the strict requirements for state immunization to allow only exemptions for medical reasons, and along this line legislators and public health professionals in almost 30 other States are working to obtain this reform (Pierik 2017). In only one year since vaccination became compulsory, the rate of vaccination in California has exceeded the vaccine safety threshold of 95% required by the WHO (Sun 2017).

Then there is the particularly interesting case of Australia, which offers financial incentives to increase the rate of recommended vaccinations: a tax deduction of Australian $129 for each child that has completed the course of vaccinations. In addition, although the country does not require from parents the compulsory presentation of a certificate for school enrolment of their children, they are not allowed to send them to school whenever the risk of epidemics appears (Walkinshaw 2011).

Lastly, there is the European context, characterized by a balanced approach. From a study carried out in 2012, of the 27 member-states of the European Union, plus Iceland and Norway, 15 do not have compulsory vaccinations, while 14 have at least one. The anti-polio vaccination is compulsory for children and adults in 12 countries, for tetanus and diphtheria in eleven and for hepatitis B in ten (Haverkate et al. 2012). Recently, the drop in vaccinations has driven France to make legal measures effective once again. On 7 January 2016, two parents who, afraid of the preservatives deemed toxic and opposed the trivalent vaccination for diphtheria, tetanus and polio for their two children, appeared in the criminal division of the court of Auxerre, in Burgundy, accused of "refusal to comply with the obligation of vaccination" and were sentenced to 2 months of imprisonment and a fine of 3750 €—French law on public health for a similar accusation entails a maximum of 6 months' imprisonment and a fine of 30,000 €. In July 2017, after an extensive debate in the French institutions on the urgency for a new vaccination policy, the French Prime

Minister announced, in the wake of the earlier Italian decision, to make 11 paediatric vaccinations compulsory in 2018, with respect to only three currently compulsory (Payet 2017).[9]

The Italian situation has changed radically in recent years. From a historical point of view, the consent or refusal of compulsory vaccinations is often linked to the perception of the risk of infection and the state of health of the population. From 1939 to the 1960s, there were the first vaccines (diphtheria, tetanus, polio) introduced by the legislator according to a principle of obligatoriness, in particular with criminal penalties for objecting parents and preventing the enrolment at school of the children without a correct vaccinal schedule. After several years of affluence and absence of major epidemics, for some time now in Italy there have been various openings for the suspension of the obligation of vaccination. The first form of decriminalization came in 1981, when the offences for the omission of vaccination were transformed into an administrative offence; the same penalty applied in 1991 for hepatitis B; the fourth and last vaccination proposed as compulsory alongside those offered as optional (measles, mumps, rubella, pertussis, HIB, meningococcus, pneumococcus, HPV, chicken pox, flu). Since 1999, all unvaccinated pupils have been allowed to attend school, and since 2001 a constitutional reform has shifted the responsibility for the organization and management of the health service, and therefore of the vaccination decisions, to the individual regional governments, generating a regional mosaic which is extremely variegated and inefficient from a health point of view. In July 2017, a law came into force that brought the number of compulsory (and free) vaccinations to ten (pertussis, HIB, measles, rubella, mumps, chicken pox, as well as the previously compulsory four), making it a requirement for school attendance by babies and children between 0 and 16. Failure to administer the compulsory vaccines entails the convocation of the parents to the local health authority to urge them to vaccinate their children and in the case of refusal—in the event that specific clinical conditions that advise against vaccination are not certified—precludes the enrolment of the children in nurseries and nursery schools, whilst failure to respect the obligation by older children entails a fine of between 100 and 500 €.

---

[9] Forster, K., *France to make vaccination mandatory from 2018*, The Independent, July 15 2017 : https://goo.gl/RZomSa ; *France plans to make 11 vaccinations compulsory for children*, The Local, 16 June 2017: https://goo.gl/LkeMXU; Children set for 11 vaccinations under new health plan, Connexion journalist, 16 June 2017: https://goo.gl/1HPFbD

# 3

# The Accusations Against Vaccinations on the Internet: Autism, Mercury and Immunological Overload

## The Conspiracy Theory on the Internet: True, False, Fictive

Data, harsh data, are the only thing that count, we could say, paraphrasing a famous quotation from Stendhal's *The Red and the Black* about the truth. At a time like the present, when we are submerged by information by media, it is not at all easy to find our way around to distinguish between what is true and what is false, in the sense of reported untruthfully or partially, or even fictive, in the sense of fake or fabricated. For my generation, which saw it come into being, the Internet has been and is a marvellous opportunity of cultural growth. Its strength lies in the freedom of the web, but so does its weakness. Alongside books and articles written by the most authoritative experts on every possible subject of human knowledge, there are texts that are cobbled together, manipulated or invented. The historian Carlo Ginzburg said this admirably in his *lectio magistralis* when he received the prestigious Balzan Prize (several of its winners have also received a Nobel Prize) in September 2011:

> Some have said that the Internet is an instrument of democracy. Taken literally, this statement is false. We have to add: it is an instrument of potential democracy. The motto of the Internet can be summarized in the words, paradoxical and politically incorrect, pronounced by Jesus: "Whoever has will be given more" (Matthew, XIII, 12). To navigate in the Internet, to distinguish the pearl from the sow's ear, you already have to have had access to culture—an access which normally (and I speak from personal experience) is associated with social privilege. The Internet, which potentially could be an instrument that could attenuate

© Springer International Publishing AG, part of Springer Nature 2018
A. Grignolio, *Vaccines: Are they Worth a Shot?*, https://doi.org/10.1007/978-3-319-68106-1_3

cultural inequalities, in the immediate, exasperates them. Schools need the Internet, of course, but the Internet, to be used according to its potential (let's say realistically one-millionth of its capacity), needs state schools that really teach.[1]

School, and in a broader sense, educating to know and the development of logical-critical skills of thinking are the only instrument that can keep us afloat in this *mare magnum* of information. Recourse to the original sources and harsh data is, therefore, the only certain evidence that we have to know whether what we have found on the Internet is true or not. However, not everybody has the instruments and the time for such philological work. Reality is different: a parent goes to the Internet to find out about vaccinations for their child and finds a series of terrifying pieces of information, which sometimes outnumber the positive ones and they cannot of course start to read articles about immunology to evaluate the reliability of the sources. This is how the doubt of the risk enters their mind and will not leave it easily.

Parents find themselves in this situation quite frequently, as shown by the studies already mentioned (Chap. 2) conducted in the United States, Canada, Australia and Italy: a fair percentage of parents decides not to vaccinate their children on the basis of information found on the Internet. This is a growing phenomenon and in a few years could be transformed into a serious national problem of public health.

There can be no doubt that the Internet often gives very bad advice as far as vaccinations are concerned because, as we will see, it collects and multiplies falsehoods and lies on the subject. However, before going on to review the best known hoaxes, we have to dwell briefly on the nature and function of the conspiracy and complot theories which are very popular on the web. The websites of "counter-information" are growing all the time and to understand this you only have to glance at the negationist sites (perhaps the most odious) which refuse the existence of the Nazi gas chambers, those that support the existence of chemical trails and naturally those against animal experimentation or vaccinations. Their uncontested growth is due to a series of reasons which we will now look at.

When support for an "alternative theory" appears on the Internet, it is impossible to imagine that the competences of the country, whether scientific, legal or humanistic, dedicate part of their energy to rejecting them. This is not how the scientific method works. Until proven otherwise, the earth is

---

[1] Carlo Ginzburg, Speech of thanks at the awards ceremony of the Balzan Prizes 2010, Milan, Fondazione Internazionale Balzan, 2011.

spherical, Italy is one of the countries with the highest life expectancy and vaccines are amongst the most effective drugs and with the best risks/benefit ratio in the world. Anyone who wants to prove that the earth is flat, that chemical trails exist that are dangerous for human health or that vaccines are ineffective or damaging is, naturally, free to do so, but they are obliged to put forward evidence, not opinions, on blogs. That the "alternative" theory is the correct one and that its approval is prevented by the scientific community is a false argument: the scientific community, before the evidence, has never prevented anything, even when the theories were innovative as in the case of Jenner or Einstein (see Chap. 4). The paradoxical nature of the "alternative theory" is served well by the "paradox of the celestial teapot" or Russell's teapot, from the name of the famous British mathematician and philosopher Bertrand Russell: he explained that the burden of proof lay upon those who intend opposing knowledge that until that moment had been confirmed by scientific evidence, and not vice versa. However, we often fall into the contrary paradox whereby, according to Russell's metaphor, someone can maintain that between the Earth and Mars there is a china teapot orbiting around the Sun, but it is so small that it cannot be detected by present-day telescopes. This "new scientific hypothesis" cannot at the moment be disproven by the scientific community, which must not doubt it a priori—showing the usual intolerable presumption—and therefore it cannot oppose funding the research. This is the typical situation of those who say, for example, that they have discovered toxic molecules in vaccines that create mental retardation or cancer. They are always invited to seek funds, through selection by public call, to prove that these substances and doses cause the etiopathology of those diseases. They are invited to do the same as all researchers, including the "revolutionary" researchers to whom they aspire, without victimization and without shortcuts: obtain funds. But these studies on alternative research are never produced because, quite simply, they do not stand up to the test of the scientific method and remain what they were originally: personal opinions not supported by reproducible empirical data that prove their validity. The scientific community cannot engage in constant duels with the counter-information on the Internet and certainly does not have the duty to use its time and money (mostly public) to prove that there are no celestial teapots between the Earth and Mars, but in the absence of discussion with the experts, counter-information spreads like wildfire.

Another reason is that conspiracy theories are more successful than scientific explanations. In general, the latter are complex and counter-intuitive, either because in comparison, conspiracy theories are comprehensible, in the sense that they reduce stress and complexity, providing a design or a series of coherent responsibilities, or because they agree with the cognitive attitude (or bias) of the finalistic perception, which tends to create connections between casual data or data without meaning (apophenia) (Kelemen et al. 2005, 2012; Kelemen and Rosset 2009). The animistic interpretation of reality is one of the most ancient and resistant strategies of adaptation and containment of environmental stress of our species, and even today when we are faced with a complex collective social fact, such as the death of the US President J.F. Kennedy, the landing on the moon, the HIV epidemic or the terrorist attack on the Twin Towers, conspiracy theories are one of the most acceptable and common explanations (Kruglanski and Webster 1996; Byford 2011; Hogg and Blaylock 2011; Bessi et al. 2015).

A number of studies also show how on the Internet, communication, especially on subjects linked to innovation such as climate change, the civilian use of nuclear power, embryonic stem cells, GMO and similar, is polarized towards extremist positions and is distributed amongst users according to a tribal logic (in clusters) based on sharing similar political–cultural values (Kahan et al. 2011; Haidt 2013). These attitudes can be ascribed both to the conspirationists and to the advocates of mainstream or scientific knowledge (Munro and Ditto 1997; Zollo et al. 2015), with the substantial difference, however, that the conspirationists show a far greater cognitive closure (Kata 2010; Wood et al. 2012; Leman and Cinnirella 2013), refusing to discuss non-conspiracy theories or visiting and commenting scientific sites (Bessi et al. 2015). Conspirationists are also more inclined towards both the "confirmation bias", which consists of looking for, selecting and interpreting only information that confirms convictions or hypotheses, and the "backfire effect" which explains why, if challenged in their beliefs with corrective scientific information, they reinforce even more their position of rejection (Lewandowsky et al. 2013; Wood et al. 2012). These biases refer to the typical dogmatic and paranoid mentality of the conspirationists (Zoja 2011), which also fosters a Manichaean vision of society—honest and authentic 'us' v. cheating and corrupt 'them'; "stay vigilant! The real numbers of the adverse reactions are kept concealed from us, they are not telling us the truth"—which not only tends to be self-reinforcing and self-fuelling, but leads to gradual civil and political disengagement (Bauer 1995; Jolley and Douglas 2013), typically represented by the rejection of the vaccinal prophylaxis.

This huge mass of discouraging data on the relationship between vaccines—but also on more general scientific subjects such as climate change—and conspiracy theories fuelled by the web is fairly homogeneous in Europe and the United States. In the case of Italy, however, another negative element is, in all probability, also at play, namely the endemic disinterest which regulates the relations between science, politics and society. Amongst the various national and international companies and institutions which measure the popularity and understanding of scientific subjects by the public, the Eurobarometer is a particularly useful instrument which has the task of cyclically assessing the "public perception of science, research and innovation" in the Member-States of the European Union. In the last observations, the Eurobarometer puts Italy as one of the countries with the lowest comprehension of the scientific method and with the lowest confidence in the ability of science to improve the quality of life, health and economic development.[2] There is more. In Italy, low scientific literacy joins—and it is a consequence of it—the high level of functional illiteracy and a relapse into illiteracy, i.e. an individual's inability to efficiently use the reading, writing and arithmetical skills that they once had, in everyday situations. These two cultural shortcomings imply a third one, reported by the summary document of the Eurispes data of 2013, which points a finger at the reduced ability of criticism by Italian society, and its "loss of the habit" of analytical doubt and calm civil discussion, which inevitably generates citizens who are "gullible" or "dogmatic".[3] The lack of these instruments of thought or of "concepts to critically understand and appreciate modernity" to use the words of the well-known Australian intelligence psychologist James R. Flynn (see Chap. 6) puts democracy at risk, because citizens (and politics) are more subject to oscillate from the radical scepticism of the conspirationists who doubt effective cures such as vaccines, to the false certainties of the quacks of the moment, who cry out about "miraculous cures" like *Stamina method* or the Hamer method. The horizon, however, is not without hope. The Observa data of 2014 indicate a clear improvement in the perception of science by Italians;[4] the minimal knowledge is also improving in that part of the population that does not inform itself of science, known as *scientific illiterates*; the channels through which the Italians are improving their scientific knowledge are increasing and being diversified and the public at scientific events and conferences is growing, while the increase in the rate of credibility towards this direct source of information and scientists is also significant.

Let us now look in brief at the main accusations against vaccines on the Internet.

---

[2] Special Eurobarometer 419, Public Perceptions of Science, Research and Innovation, Report, October 2014, http://tinyurl.com/jnrhnbt

[3] Eurispes. 25° Rapporto Italia 2013. Documento di Sintesi, http://tinyurl.com/k4wwe4q

[4] Annuario Scienza e Tecnologia e Società 2014: edizione speciale decennale. Dieci anni di scienza nella società, a cura di Massimiano Bucchi e Barbara Saracino, Il Mulino, Bologna 2014, http://tinyurl.com/ojwwvek

# The Economic Criticisms: Multinational Corporations and Patents

The economic interests, which in principle could have come under the category of "ideological reasons", are perhaps the commonest accusation against vaccinations, to the point that it is even raised by those who are not contrary to vaccinations (Greenberg et al. 2017). The criticism of the economic interests underlying the spread of vaccines is made in different ways (Corbellini 2013; Offit 2015; Reich 2016), but the central idea is that they are not necessary or are not safe, and that the only reason why today, in a society without infectious diseases, they are produced and distributed to the whole population is due to the interests of the pharmaceutical multinational corporations, grouped together under the generally disparaging name of Big Pharma.

This accusation is also inevitably extended to scientists, researchers, doctors and healthcare operators, who are all alleged to be accomplices in keeping quiet about the uselessness or the harmfulness of vaccines, because they are in the pay of the pharmaceutical industry. Let's try and see how things really stand.

The pharmaceutical industry is no different from all other industries. It invests money to create products that it then has to sell on the market to continue in business. This is what car manufacturers, mobile phone and computer manufacturers and even the food industry, including the organic one, do. There is no sector, as it is a human activity and therefore fallible, that is free from occasional scandals or excesses in the name of profit. In free market democracies, it is right that the guilty, if judged so at a trail, pay for the offences committed, but to accuse the whole of the pharmaceutical industry, especially the part devoted to developing vaccines, is unreasonable and prejudicial, for a number of important reasons.

In the first place, unlike car manufacturers and IT companies for example, pharmaceutical companies produce drugs that improve or save millions of human lives. In this sense, the reasoning could even be overturned. Looking at pure empirical data, it is at the least curious that nobody ever takes the trouble of publicly thanking the pharmaceutical companies for the fact that in the past century they have given—thanks to antibiotics, vaccines, painkillers and, more recently, mood stabilizers, monoclonal antibodies and lifesaving drugs against cancer, HIV and cardiovascular diseases—a decisive contribution to the improvement and lengthening of life after centuries of diseases and physical pain. We all have a very strong bond with our mobile phone, but the difference between a phone call and a drug that can save your life or relieve a stabbing pain or feelings of suicide is incommensurable. In general, there is great admiration for the two main companies that make mobile phones: Steve Jobs, especially after his premature death, is considered a planetary guru. But we would all be in difficulty if we had to say which pharmaceutical company had just put on to the market the drug that in a few days eradicates a pathogenic agent that has been a scourge for humans for at least five centuries, the virus of hepatitis C. This is a terrible infectious disease that in the world affects from 130 to 170 million individuals (one million in Italy alone) and which in 2013 was responsible for 700,000 deaths from cirrhosis and liver cancer, which can be traced to it. Therefore, scandals and corruption in companies being equal, we could in theory be more indulgent towards pharmaceutical companies due to the well-being that their products have produced for humanity in the last century and a half. On the contrary, there is a widespread feeling of mistrust of them and the erroneous conviction that it is a particularly dishonest and venal field—the anti-hepatitis drug has been put on the market in some countries at a price considered high but, beyond the need to better regulate the mechanisms of price auctions, the costs/benefits always have to be weighed up, i.e. the cost of the drug compared with the lifelong cost of a chronic hepatitis patient. This mistaken perception, which is willingly echoed by some media, means that the harshest and most lasting criticisms coagulate around their common corporate unlawful actions. It would be ridiculous, as well as liable to accusation of the same ideology, even though in the opposite way, to defend pharmaceutical companies automatically or to treat them as victims. Absolutely not. The pharmaceutical companies have to be treated like all the others and, above all, for what they are: companies based on innovation that have to reinvest a (substantial) part of their (high) profits to finance (expensive) research for new or better products.

The erroneous social perception of which they are the object is linked to an expectation, equally erroneous, about their profits: the curious expectation that they must have an inclination for charity, by virtue of the fact that they deal with health. This is the first criticism that arises as soon as a pharmaceutical company negotiates the purchase price of a new drug with the national regulatory agencies or when the Ministry of Health purchases the supplies of vaccines for seasonal flu: discounts or lower prices are claimed or the demand is that they are supplied free of charge. Nobody asks an engineer to be charitable, we do not even ask those who produce staple goods for survival such as food to be charitable and of course we do not ask Apple for free iPhones and, looking closely, we do not even ask healthcare operators to work for charity. Psychologists, psychiatrists, nurses, clinicians and surgeons, including those who offer "alternative" treatments not based on evidence of efficacy, are all paid, according to the market rules of supply and demand. This reasoning, however obvious it may be, is suspended when it comes to evaluating the work of pharmaceutical companies; moreover, their donations for social, educational and health projects are in general the largest, in 2010 having reached the maximum ever (according to "Forbes"). In the specific case of vaccines, the pharmaceutical companies give such a high number to developing countries that genuine international supply chains have been created, regulated by the UNICEF/WHO Vaccine Donation Guidelines and by the GAVI Vaccine Alliance[5]—even though a great deal remains to be done to reduce the time between when a new vaccine is put on to the market in the West and its donation to countries in greatest need of it. The subject of the profit on drugs, of waiving the rules of the market and gratuitousness, however senseless it may be, is very present on the Internet; the critics of Big Pharma though should abide by the same criterion, for example, by giving up a substantial part of their salaries, or selling their products at a loss for humanitarian purposes, according to the old (Kantian) moral rule whereby it is good practice to be the first to submit to the rule that you want to impose on others.

Nor do the critical groups that populate the Internet take into account an essential economic element which is often ignored: pharmaceutical research is very expensive and time-consuming. In the first place, multidisciplinary and highly specialized work groups have to be formed that study promising molecules; then on average it takes 12 years for research to become a drug available on the market. Lastly, consider that the starting point is the analysis of a number of molecules that goes from between 5000 and 10,000 to succeed in obtaining a drug of proven efficacy, all for an average cost of between five hundred million and one billion euro. This tortuous process, as is obvious, aims at protecting patients, with continuous trials divided into three preclinical stages and no less than two and a half years of analysis by the national public regulatory agency (FDA), which analyses in the tiniest detail the validity of the data provided before approving the drug for marketing (Douglas and Samant 2017). It is indispensable that proceeds from patents come into this process, but there is also a great deal of misunderstanding on this subject, verging on "cognitive dissonance". This is the situation in which an individual has contrasting beliefs and opinions, which activate incoherent behaviour and are a cause of emotional distress and which are, therefore, denied or justified artificially. For example, it is the case of an individual who says he hates thieves

---

[5] GAVI, launched in 2000, is a partnership of public and private subjects—WHO, UNICEF, World Bank, Bill & Melinda Gates Foundation, etc.—with the aim of improving access to immunization for the populations of poor countries. See in particular the Vaccine Donation Policy, http://tinyurl.com/h4sze3y

and at the same time buys a bicycle or mobile phone at knock-down prices on the black market, without checking their dubious origin.

Let's take the case of ABS, a mechanism which is now installed on all cars to allow braking more efficiently, depending on the slipperiness of the road surface: it is a very useful patent, and nobody complains about it when they buy a car; on the contrary, everybody wants it. The same applies to the airbag, the soles of many technical shoes or our mobile phones and the thousands of applications that are downloaded every day. It also applies to food: people who like apples, like me, cannot fail to know the very good Pink Lady apples; well, they are patented and they have not altered the market or impoverished farmers. Fuji apples, Zespri Gold and Kamut flour, greatly loved by vegans and by those who buy "organic" food, are also covered by patents. Patents and royalties are nothing but a form of protection to guarantee for the producer who has invested and risked money—money which the state, especially in the case of very costly drugs, could not have—to ensure an economic return. In addition, the pharmacological patents have a duration of 20 years, and 1 year from when they are filed they can already be reworked and improved by other researchers in order to allow open competition for the development of an innovation. People tear their hair out over the patents and proceeds on lifesaving drugs and vaccines but ignore those for mobiles, cars and Kamut flour: in this sense, it is reasonable to see these criticisms as the result of cognitive dissonance or an ethical "double standard". As well as being amongst the safest drugs (as we will see in Chap. 5), vaccines are also the most inexpensive (on average the price is between 20 and 30 €) and, therefore, with a very low impact coming from the patent. This is also without counting that for over 90% of vaccines, the intellectual property and the patents date back more than 12 years and today have expired. More, in general, in this case too, the numerous humanitarian and philanthropic examples of waiving the patent to reduce the price and reach the highest number of people are ignored. Jonas Salk (1914–1995) who in 1955 produced the first vaccine against polio—with an estimated value at the time of $7 billion—waived the patent and so did his colleague Albert Sabin (1906–1993) with another longer lasting vaccine against polio. Suspending the economic interests on the vaccines, even making them free of charge (therefore much more than waiving the patent) has also been seen in very recent cases: for example, a well-known pharmaceutical company donated the HPV vaccine against cervical cancer to an African country for 3 years, while during the Ebola epidemic, the Canadian health agency that was developing the vaccine, still at the experimental stage, decided to donate, against a strong international regulation, the supplies available for the vast African population affected.

Before going on to the other arguments, it is worthwhile dealing with two other criticisms on the economic level. We regularly read on the Internet that in order to become rich with vaccines, the pharmaceutical multinational corporations are alleged to fan excessive fears about infectious diseases and according to some sites they even cause their spread. This argument does not stand up in theory or in practice. A simple, but unprejudiced, mental experiment can be of help: if we were to take the Managing Director of a pharmaceutical company and deprive him of every moral value, so that he acts like the cold calculator who chooses the corporate policy solely on the grounds of income, and we were to ask him to find a strategy to increase turnover, his answer should be: "Let's stop producing vaccines, because with a product of 10 or 20 € we offer the population immunity for life against terrible diseases which, between pharmacological treatment and hospital care of a few hundred infected patients, would give us incomparably higher earnings". This is a nonsensical thought, but it is the overturned reasoning that the conspirationists propose and which explains well how vaccines absolutely do not generate great earnings. To understand the numbers at stake, it is sufficient to give some concrete figures: an interesting study of health economics which examined the average expenditure in the countries of the European Union for the costs of treatment of a single tuberculosis (TBC) patient in 2011 indicates a cost of 10,282 € for every form of infection sensitive to pharmacological treatment, 57,213 € for every multi-resistant infection and 170,744 € for every tubercular treatment with high resistance to pharmacological therapies, for a total of 536 million euro, against an average cost of about 30 € for a Calmette-Guérin vaccine which gives lifelong protection from TBC (Diel et al. 2014). In another case, it has been estimated, based on WHO data, that the gradual eradication of smallpox between 1978 and 1997 meant, at worldwide level, a saving of $168 billion. This is a massive amount of money that has been saved (without counting the lives and human suffering) which otherwise would have gone into the coffers of the health services and companies manufacturing drugs and health machinery.[6] This reasoning, clearly, applies to all the great epidemics, like smallpox, polio, measles and the plague, which have affected millions of people, whose treatment would have yielded astronomical figures which were eradicated at the ridiculous cost of a vial of vaccine. One interesting study has calculated in the United States the annual economic cost, paid by all the taxpayers, associated with the health expenditure due to infectious diseases preventable by vaccination: in 2015, the cost was of $8.95 billion.

---

[6] United States General Accounting Office, *Infectious Diseases. Analysis of Eradication or Elimination Estimates*, 1998, p. 9: https://www.hsdl.org/?view&did=487464

People who were not vaccinated are responsible for at least 80% of this expenditure, i.e. $7.1 billion (Ozawa et al. 2016). It is curious that those who maintain that there is a great and hidden economic operation behind the distribution or imposition of vaccines have never looked at the data. One recent study in six important European countries (Germany, England, France, Italy, Spain, Portugal and Switzerland) shows that none exceed 0.5% of the budget of the National Health Services for vaccinations and although all the countries (with the exception of Spain) have annually increased their health expenditure, with France at an annual rate of 2.6% (time span 2008–2013) and the United Kingdom at 8.1% (2008–2012), the cost of vaccines has always dropped: −6.2% in Germany (2008–2014), −6.7% in Spain (2008–2012), −4.2% in France (2008–2013) (Ethgen et al. 2016). These data confirm that not only do the decisions of the unvaccinated have a negative impact on the rest of society, both at biological level and economic level, but that the perspective according to which it is the economic interests of the multinationals that govern the sector of vaccinations is unreasonable.

Furthermore, not many people know that the net balance between research, production and sale of the vaccinations is so negligible that many pharmaceutical multinationals are abandoning the sector because it is not very profitable. Today only five major pharmaceutical companies produce the majority of the vaccinations, while in 1980 there were 17 and in 1967 26 (Offit 2005). Consider, for example, the last great epidemic which frightened the whole world, the spread of the Ebola virus in West Africa in 2014. The two vaccines approved by the US regulatory agency, the FDA, were developed by two entities not linked to the major pharmaceutical companies. One was developed by the Public Health Agency of Canada, which then granted the licence to NewLink Genetics, a small American biotech firm, and subsequently to Merck & Co.; the other one was created by a small Italian biotech company, Okairos, which then in part sold it to the British pharmaceutical company GlaxoSmithKline (see Chap. 5). In the case of Ebola as in other vaccines for other infectious diseases, the major groups do not invest because, as there is not a large economic return, they prefer to leave the research for innovative vaccines to small biotech firms, so that they are the ones who take the risk in developing effective and promising remedies which, in the case of success, are possibly funded or even acquired by the large groups. Reality is not, however, always as rosy as in the fortunate case of Ebola, and the research and creativity of small or medium-sized research centres is not always necessarily capable of finding such prompt solutions. Considering the costs and time of developing drugs, it is very much to be hoped that the pharmaceutical multinational corporations continue to produce and invest in research in vaccines.

The last argument concerns the supposed connivance and corruption of doctors and healthcare operators, deemed to be in the pay of the multinationals, in fostering the spread of vaccines. It ignores that biomedical research is a transparent global competition, where all the researchers, at all latitudes, can take part with their contributions offering public and certifiable data. In the specific case, for example, in which it is believed that vaccine X causes autism, it is inconceivable that at least one of the hundreds of thousands of researchers in the world has not been able to publish a single shred of proof that supports the international parameters and proves this relationship. The conspiracy, although well organized, cannot by definition include 100% of the experts of a given sector, but only a small percentage of influential figures—otherwise, instead of a complot and conspiracy, it would be a public agreement. In this case too, reality proves the inconsistency of a similar way of reasoning. The interesting fact is that now and again some researcher throws down the gauntlet of challenge hypothesizing, for example, the relationship between autism and vaccines, and the rest of the community checks the data and proves their falsity, just as in the Wakefield case. This is why, to date, those who accuse vaccines have been mocked as "charlatans" in search of publicity or interested in selling their "alternative" products (as illustrated in Chap. 4).

Lastly, more harsh data from reality: in the United States, of the 22 medical specializations, paediatricians—the medical category that most undersigns vaccines—oscillate between the third last and the last position concerning the amount of their salary (the most affluent are orthopaedists and cardiologists).[7] If, as part of the Internet maintains, there were a ton of money flowing from the multinationals towards the doctors who prescribe the vaccines, they would certainly not be languishing at the bottom of the ranking.

## The Logical Errors: Principle of Precaution and Balance of Information

There is also a category of logical errors which is fairly full. The mother of all the misundertstandings on vaccines, focus on which would be sufficient to take apart the whole accusation for all the paediatric diseases that they are suspected of causing, is the confusion between causation and temporal correlation. In other words, the vaccines are suspected of "causing" autism, neurological diseases or immune pathologies because they "temporally correlate"

---

[7] *Medscape Physicians Compensation Report 2014*, http://tinyurl.com/zw5dtso; "Washington Post", 18 April 2014; Pam Tobey, *Doctors Still Make Good Money*, http://tinyurl.com/hbktlg3

with the vaccinal calendar, i.e. they appear in the same period (between 3 and 15–24 months). Let us look at why two events which take place in the same period of time can be independent.

The diseases of the immune system generally appear with weaning, a process where there is high immune stimulation due both to the entrance of a broad spectrum of new molecules delivered by food, after months of the mother's milk, and to the development of the intestinal bacterial flora (the so-called *microbiome*), a set of several thousands of different species of "good" microorganisms that are (as symbionts) in the human digestive tube, helping digestion and protecting it from infections. The genes of these microorganisms of the intestinal flora—equal to one hundred times the number of genes of the human genome, a fact which makes some researcher say that they are super-organisms (organisms that host other organisms) and the proteins they produce establish cross-talk made up of reciprocal stimulations with the immune system of the human host (see Chap. 5). In the event that there were a predisposition of an already latent pathology, these numerous antigenic stimulations due to weaning, which coincide in time with the first cycle of vaccines, would bring out the immune diseases. The same temporal correlation applies to the greatest suspect of vaccines, the trivalent MMR: it is administered between the 13th and 15th month of life, therefore in the phase of cognitive development when children start to say their first phrases and establish more interactive and playful forms of relations with their parents and with objects. It is only at this time that the parents may notice any suspicious attitudes (including the typical one of lining up the objects) which reveal possible symptoms of autism. Numerous studies, some of which emerged to prove the falsity of Wakefield's accusation of autism (see the next paragraph), prove that it is a temporal correlation, and that autism appears with the same frequency and in the same period of time both in vaccinated children and in children who have not been vaccinated (as will be seen below, in this chapter). These and many other data show beyond any doubt that autism and vaccinations take place in the same period of time (therefore they are correlated) and that there is no causal nexus between them.

There are many events that are correlated without one being the cause of the other, just as there are many statistical instruments that can establish whether there is a causal nexus between two variables that do not appear in the same period of time or that seem independent. The Internet is full of resources, and alongside the conspirationists there are also professional debunkers, who get fun out of unmasking falsities, exaggerated assertions and quackeries.

In this regard, there is a diagram that circulates widely in the Internet which "proves" how in the United States there was a very close correlation in the period 2006–2011 between the drop in the murder rate (from 17,200 to 14,700) and the drop (same numbers) in the diffusion of Internet Explorer, the well-known Internet browser, gradually replaced by the more efficient Chrome: naturally this is fictitious evidence, as revealed by the ironic conclusion in the caption under the diagram: "Prevent murders, choose Chrome!" During the terrible polio epidemic which in the first decades of the twentieth century spread in the United States, social psychosis practised looking for the weirdest causes, accusing cats (in 1916 in New York 70,000 were eliminated), bilberries, Italian immigrants, milk and even sugar—a lesson to bear in mind today as well. In 1940 the doctor Benjamin Sandler published an article in the scientific journal "The American Journal of Pathology" in which he hypothesized that an alteration of the metabolism of carbohydrates, and in particular a low level of sugar in the blood (hypoglycaemia), made laboratory animals and humans more susceptible to infections by the polio virus (Sandler 1941). In order to avoid variations of the metabolic effects of sugars, the first to be banned from diets were ice creams: in the newspapers of the time (and in the current reconstruction on the Internet) diagrams were diffused, apparently unequivocal which "proved" the perfect correlation between the sale of ice creams and the incidence of polio, including in consideration of the fact that the highpoints of the epidemics took place in the summer, when there was the greatest consumption of ice cream. Recently a scientific article published in 2012 in the authoritative scientific journal "New England Journal of Medicine" asked, with elegant irony and very accurate calculations, whether the consumption of chocolate (a food rich in a type of flavonoids capable of increasing cognitive performances and slowing down mental ageing) in a population could be correlated with its average intelligent quotient, as the highest number of Nobel prize-winners come from countries characterized by a high consumption of chocolate, such as Switzerland, Sweden, the United Kingdom and the United States (Messerli 2012).

Those who do not have basic knowledge in the field of statistics—not very common in the anti-vaccine portals, it would seem—find it very difficult to find their way around in these arguments. These are the consequences of that historical innovation which was mentioned in the first paragraph and which continues through the whole book with various questions, and to which we will return in the conclusions: for the first time in the history of the evolution of our species, the whole population has the chance to have free access to documents on health that include the concept of risk, and that are difficult to interpret because they are for (and written by) experts of the sector who know how to manage and weigh cognitively complex information: multifactor causes, calculations on the risks/benefits ratio, probability uncertainty, contradictory messages. Our brain, as it has been selected by evolution for other tasks, often responds in a disadaptive or inefficient way to this information. We have already seen how our cognitive apparatus is influenced by the finalistic bias: this tends to create connections between data that are not correlated. It is therefore easy to imagine how strong the finalistic temptation is in the case in which the events include, as in the case of the trivalent vaccine and autism, a simple (but casual) temporal correlation. For our brain, it is an irresistible temptation, but which often leads to error.

In the biomedical field, these concordances appear in even more complex contexts, and therefore it becomes difficult to analyse the causes of a pathology. For example, the concept of the "confounding factor", a situation in which one or more factors, other than those which are the object of the research, are responsible for the association which we have observed, distorting the interpretation of the data, eludes outsiders. If, for example, it is discovered that a population that lives close to a repeater has a greater incidence of tumours (the Internet has also debated this at length), it cannot be taken for granted that the waves of the repeater are the cause. Indeed, in many cases, after epidemiological studies on the surrounding community, it is proven that, for example, it includes a home for the elderly, which makes the rate of mortality and cancer of that population rise, or that there is another toxic factor, such as polluted ground water. Coffee was also unjustly accused for years of being the cause of heart attacks, before understanding that between the heart attack and coffee there were many other confounding factors that had not been analysed in the studies but which were correlated to coffee drinkers—such as smoking, the decrease in the number of hours of sleep, and the alteration of the sleep-wakefulness circadian cycle.

As the state of health is a multifactorial factor, i.e. it depends on genetic predisposition and on a complex series of cultural and environmental factors, the frequent alarming messages launched by the Internet, in which hasty relations are established between mortality rates and various forms of environmental pollution, have to be taken with a pinch of salt. For example, as we will see shortly, the naturist prejudice, which comes under the ideological errors, is very frequent in the blogs of anti-vaccinationists: for naturists, urban life, full of pollutants, stress and "artificial" chemical-pharmacological treatments, weakens the organism, especially the immune system of children, unlike a "natural" lifestyle, which is capable of recovering the habits of our "grandparents' days" when the diet was based on "organic" food, and drugs and medicines—and naturally vaccines as well—were not used. As we have already seen on several occasions, science is often counter-intuitive and some recent North American epidemiological data tell us that in the metropolises the population on average lives longer—there are for example more hospitals and doctors per number of inhabitants—with respect to country-dwellers where the rate of obesity and smoking is higher. The mental state cannot be that idyllic either, considering that the suicide rate in young people is much higher than in the cities (Singh and Siahpush 2014; Fontanella et al. 2015).

Another logical error common on the anti-vaccination sites is the difference between *ex ante* and *ex post* evaluations, i.e. evaluations made before or after the facts have happened. These are two Latin expressions introduced in the 1930s, by the economists of the Stockholm School, to indicate the programmed or foreseen level of a given economic variable (*ex ante*) and to distinguish it from the assumed or achieved one (*ex post*). It has to be said that *ex ante* analyses concern uncertain variables, and therefore the evaluations relative to them consist of distributions of probability, or estimates mainly based on data collected in the past, whereas in the *ex post* analyses the data is, or should be, certain. When the government has to take a political decision on seasonal vaccinations, it has to make *ex ante* decisions: often the anti-vaccinationists and sometimes some media ignore this delicate difference and denounce agreements between public health professionals and pharmaceutical companies, maintaining that the number of batches of vaccines and the relative expenditure were excessive, because at the end of the season there has been no significant pandemic. This is a gross logical error: you do not evaluate "in hindsight" something that can probabilistically only be decided before the events. It would be like concluding that safety belts or helmets are useless every time that we see people who do not use them arrive safe and sound at their destination. When a season starts, the experts do not know how dangerous the flu that is coming is the degree of efficacy of the vaccine and other unforeseeable environmental factors (such as the fluctuations in temperature). The people in charge of health policies have to take decisions in a context of great uncertainty and make a complex analysis of the risks/benefits ratio. The fact that some years there remain batches that are not used is the sign of a mild flu and a virus kept under control, precisely by a vast vaccinal cover. It is difficult to foresee the outbreaks of epidemics, and it must not be forgotten that epidemics of flu such as "Spanish flu" which caused between 50 and 100 million deaths after the First World War (see Chap. 5) may return.

Two other fairly significant mistaken assumptions circulate online. The first concerns a mistaken perception of the risk. This is an issue which, as we will see, refers to the "principle of precaution". Essentially, the subject of the risk deems that it is sensible to avoid vaccines as they have caused a certain number of ascertained cases of severe side effects. The wrong assumption underlying this subject can be understood by reversing the reasoning with a question: do any medical treatments with a zero risk exist? Absolutely no. It is difficult to accept it, but ours is not a society with a zero risk. Indeed, as will be discussed in the conclusive chapter, the perception of risk is a topic destined to occupy an increasingly central role in today's knowledge society (Gigerenzer 2015). In the knowledge society, citizens, through the development of various forms of direct, deliberative and participative democracy, will increasingly often be called on to reckon with complex health, financial and professional decisions. We are at risk when we go to work by car, we risk in love and in money and we take a risk every time we eat a new food. Even introducing a lot of water all of a sudden into the body (after prolonged stress or in post-operative induced hydration), we put our life in danger, risking acute intoxication from water. Naturally, we also take a risk when we take any drug, vaccines included.

As the zero degree of risk does not exist and, on the contrary, absolutely everything entails risk, the only rational approach in the face of biomedical treatment is to weigh up the risks and benefits of the individual treatment and then compare them with the risks and benefits of other competing treatments or other daily actions. Aspirin is perhaps the best known and commonest drug in the world, which can be bought in pharmacies without a prescription, but it also entails risks: like all drugs in its category (NSAIDs, non-steroidal anti-inflammatory drugs) such as analgesics, antipyretics and anti-inflammatories, if used improperly it can cause severe side effects. In Spain, NSAIDs and aspirin kill 15.3 people out of 100,000 patients who use them for prolonged periods of time (Lanza et al. 2009) and in the United States the deaths increase to 310, for a total of 16,500 deaths annually and 76,000 hospitalizations of serious cases, for cardiovascular and gastrointestinal diseases such as ulcers, haemorrhages and kidney and liver failure (Singh and Triadafilopoulos 1999). Yet there are no Internet sites dedicated to anti-aspirin and anti-NSAIDs movements nor are there VIPs who cry out about a world conspiracy. Here, we are not advising against a drug: it is worth clarifying that aspirin and NSAIDs are extremely effective drugs and with effects that are mainly beneficial. In the West every year, on average, eighty tablets are consumed per person; like all pharmacological treatments, however, they must be taken with moderation. The intention is rather to suggest a comparison between two medicines (the commonest and the most feared), to realize that our brain "crashes" when it has to deal with choices that concern risk and probability. The same parent who refuses to give their child a vaccination gives them an aspirin or NSAID without any qualms. On average, there is only one adverse effect every million doses of vaccine, whereas prolonged use of NSAIDs can cause death with a probability that is 1500 times greater or cause a severe allergic (anaphylactic) shock—therefore with the same effect and with a single dose as in the vaccine—in one person out of 50,000 (coming second after penicillin, as a category of drugs with a high risk of anaphylactic shock). This risk is, therefore, twenty times greater than with a vaccine (Berkes 2003; Marx 2010). If the ratio between risks and benefits is then analysed, it is even more paradoxical: while the vaccine saves a life from severe infectious, often fatal, diseases, and which put the whole community at risk, aspirin and NSAIDs relieve minor disorders.

This widespread incapacity to evaluate the real risks, which on the Internet reaches its maximum expression, inevitably results in an indiscriminate and inhibiting feeling of fear which takes the name of "principle of precaution". In its most radical form, it maintains that, as we do not have absolute certainty (zero risk) about a given technological or scientific innovation, it is better to block its development and spread by way of precaution. Those supporting it pander to a cautionary policy in regard to innovations which a part of society, but hardly ever the experts of the sector, deems "controversial", especially regarding future or long-lasting developments on the health of the population. If based on empirical and epidemiological analyses which evaluate studies of the impact on statistical samples, on a real examination of the risks and of the benefits, as well as in a comparison of the risks with the alternatives available that can reach the same benefits, the principle of precaution becomes a useful and effective instrument. Unfortunately, on the Internet, it is used only as a rhetorical instrument to fuel irrational fears and create the fear of interests of dark lobbies of power. To understand the risks of a similar use of the principle of precaution, a simple mental experiment is sufficient, in which all the most important techno-scientific innovations of the last two centuries and their possible risks are reviewed. We realize immediately that with the logic of "zero risk" or the "possible long-lasting harmful risks", we would still be in the Stone Age. The discovery of fire gave humans enormous advantages, from warmth to cooking food, to sterilization, but it entails evident risks that are still present today. Nobody today would give up the advantages of an apartment with gas and electricity, but a system of underground electricity and gas pipes without a doubt entails some risks. Even a car can be a terrible instrument of death if driven at high speed into an innocent crowd, but instead of banning cars, it has been useful to establish agreed rules on using them and penalties for those who do not abide by them. On the fears of long-lasting effects—which as we will see in the next chapter is one of the war horses of the quacks—we only have to highlight here that, from a historical point of view, catastrophist attitudes have always, and systematically, been wrong. At the end of the nineteenth century, it was thought that the dung from carriage horses would have invaded the streets of the large cities; then cars running on petrol arrived. In the middle of the 1950s, it was thought that nuclear energy would have taken humanity towards the nuclear holocaust whereas today it is a source of energy greatly used in technologically advanced countries and many, overall, deem it less polluting than fossil coal. Then there was the fear of a pandemic of AIDS, imagining apocalyptic scenarios and divine punishments, but in 20 years, scientific research has put antiviral treatments on the market which have multiplied by five the life expectancy of a patient in the late 1980s. Those who appeal to the principle of precaution to refuse vaccinations, therefore, are only "throwing the baby out with the bathwater", revealing that they have a cognitive incapacity to work out the risk.

The last logical error concerns so-called balanced scientific information, i.e. the equality of conditions on the level of visibility in the media and in politics for a theory deemed "controversial". In the last few decades, this circumstance has put at serious risk the credibility of the Italian health institutions. When a scientific debate arises—think of climate change, evolutionism or the relationship between autism and vaccines—politics and the news media tend to imagine a debate during which "both sides have to be heard". This debate, thinking of the theories of the anti-vaccinationists or the "alternative" cures for cancer, opposes the community of experts with committees and associations of relatives of patients, VIPs and, as is obvious, those directly concerned, the inventors of the alternative therapy, without any validated scientific evidence but, in total conflict of interest, with miraculous cures to be sold (see Chap. 4). Fuelled by the news media, the debate grows and public opinion is divided between those who are for and those who are against, while protests in the streets ask politics for the freedom of treatment and to be able to use (subsidized by the State) the alternative therapies as *compassionate treatments.* Television programmes and the press devote in-depth discussions and articles to the issue and politicians are asked to make a decision, at times establishing committees of inquiry. At this point, in general, the logic collapses and the country runs aground in the shallows of demagogy and irrationality. Politicians and the media, with some significant exceptions, instead of asking for explanations from the greatest experts on the subject in order to evaluate the validity and reliability of the data supporting the "alternative" therapy, worry about impartiality or the fair balance of mutually opposed views. This situation leads to what is known as a false balance, a typical cognitive bias of some journalists that emerges when they present opposing points of view as equal, with only one based on scientific evidence. On television and in the interviews in the newspapers, alongside scientists and experts, there appear people who do not have the slightest idea of what a controlled clinical trial is to evaluate the efficacy of a pharmacological therapy, but who, to make up for this, tell of personal experiences of treatment or invoke the therapeutic freedom of the patient (at the expense of the citizens) or the absence of treatment available in traditional medicine and therefore the right to use compassionate treatments. In this way, there is the impression that the debate is balanced because "both sides of the discussion" are present. Nothing could be more wrong!

If in the place of a therapy we choose the case of the solar system, the paradox immediately becomes clear. Let's imagine that a researcher announces having found an innovative method to prove that it is the Sun that goes around the Earth and not vice versa, as traditional science would have us believe. After all—this is the thesis of the alternative theory—the intuition of man and his feelings, which are based on direct observation and common sense have suggested for thousands of years that it is the Sun that rotates around the Earth. What do we do in this case? Do we air TV programmes based on impartiality and balanced information, in which on the one hand there are those who defend the traditional heliocentric system and on the other those who support the new alternative geocentric theory, with the Earth in the centre? Do we publish articles in the press that present a correct perspective, because it is based on two opinions being compared? Then a new researcher pops up who maintains, but the data are not yet final, that the Earth is flat. Do we have to compare the two theories in this case as well? And if there were parliamentary questions or requests for clarification by politicians—perhaps to correct or supplement school textbooks, as was attempted against Darwin's theory of evolution—are hearings organized with the representatives of the two theories? Of course not. Balanced information does not exist in science: evidence proves that the earth is round and that it is the Sun that is at the centre of our planetary system. It is a theory corroborated by facts that have been repeated and are repeatable and therefore anyone who believes that the trivalent MMR vaccine causes autism, anyone who imagines that there are toxic excipients of metals that lead to neurological diseases and anyone who suspects that combined vaccines like the trivalent or hexavalent ones established in the vaccinal calendar weaken the immune system, facilitate the development of autoimmune diseases or cancer, has to prove it with facts and not opinions or personal experiences. However, the opponents of vaccines including that insignificant percentage of doctors (0.03%, see the next chapter) use opinions, hearsay and personal experience that confirm these theories. Equal conditions in a scientific debate are granted to two theories corroborated by facts and experiments validated by international procedures and published in scientific journals, whereas interviews, television programmes and web pages are not sufficient to prove that a theory is valid and, therefore, worthy of equal treatment in the media. The scientific method came into being precisely to stem the age-old mistakes that healers, naturists and doctors, often in good faith, made when self-evaluating the efficacy of their treatments.

The obligation of being based on proven facts is perhaps what distinguishes science from the humanistic disciplines, where opinions have greater importance and it is therefore sensible to invoke equal conditions of discussion. In this case too, however, without ever derogating from evidence, otherwise the paradoxical and unacceptable situation is reached where, to give a historical example, proof of the existence of the gas chambers, accepted by 99.99% of historians—and based on enormous amounts of data that are coherent and continuously rechecked and updated—takes on the same dignity as the manipulations of data offered by a small group of negationists in search of visibility (Ginzburg 2006). This idea of relativism (a philosophical position which denies the existence of objective truths, considered arbitrary) is not only theoretically incorrect, but socially harmful: the data of reality cannot be either marginalized or rejected (Grignolio 2015). Furthermore, in the public debate conducted by the media, sooner or later the effective difference between fact and opinion will have to be confronted (Jervis 2014). If it is true that scientific facts have different levels of certainty, and that scientific theories are not free of interpretations, it is also true that in science interpretations are not infinite and above all, they are not all the same. Some are true, some need to be tested, others are false and are rejected. As ideas are not all true, not everyone is right, consequently especially in the decisions aimed at reaching the common good which influence the political life of citizens (medical therapies, vaccines, etc.) not all positions have the same right of citizenship. Everyone, of course, is free to express their opinion and defend their beliefs, but only the ideas evaluated by competent people and supported by data and reliable evidence according to international standards can be taken into consideration in the public debate and by political decision makers.

## False or Manipulated Reconstructions: Autism

Let's start by dealing with autism and the Wakefield case, but first a warning is necessary for some readers. It has been experimentally proven that those parents who are totally contrary to paediatric vaccinations, believed responsible for causing autism, even when shown the evidence, the data and proof that acquit vaccinations once and for all, do not change their minds about their dangerousness. These parents even show that they understand the data perfectly well yet they persevere in their refusal to vaccinate their children

(Nyhan et al. 2014). If they happen to read these lines, they should not waste any time, skip them and go straight to the last chapter, in which some possible, recent solutions to overcome their cognitive refusal are suggested (Chap. 6).

Falsification, fabrication and plagiarism: these are the three possible forms of fraud in science (Bucci 2015), whether they are perpetrated by scientists or by improvized and anonymous "experts" on vaccines present on the Internet. *Fabrication* refers to the artificial construction of data or an image, *falsification* the choice or selective omission of only the necessary data, often deliberately assembled, to prove the validity of their research and, lastly, *plagiarism* refers to appropriation through completely or partially copying someone else's data or research—obviously this appropriation has to be distinguished from the lawful, even extensive, use of someone else's data through the open acknowledgement in bibliographical references.

The most famous case of fraud by falsification concerning vaccines is without any doubt the association between the trivalent vaccine and autism, created by the British surgeon and gastroenterologist Andrew Wakefield in 1998. This is a blatant case which popped up in the media all over the world and for which England is still paying very dearly. As has already been said, 20 years earlier, the United Kingdom had already been the scene of a social phobia against the pertussis vaccine, originated by the mystification by some anti-vaccination groups based on the documents of London's Great Ormond Street Hospital. This was an event outside the scientific world, and the health authorities reacted energetically through the media, as well as circulating an extensive and targeted national study which denied any relationship between the pertussis vaccine and the onset of neurological diseases (as described in Chap. 2). The Wakefield affair is more complicated, because in this case the spark that started the blaze, which has still not died down, was an event perceived as inside the scientific community, namely an article written by a doctor, Andrew Wakefield, together with twelve other colleagues, in one of the most important and authoritative scientific journals in the world, "The Lancet". Let's look at the facts.

Between July 1996 and February 1997, at the Royal Free Hospital in London, Wakefield analysed a small sample of 12 children (average age of 6) who had received the trivalent MMR vaccination about 10 days earlier: in 8 of them he found signs of the autistic spectrum and symptoms of intestinal inflammation, which he renamed *autistic enterocolitis* (Wakefield et al. 1998). The association of these three events—trivalent vaccine, intestinal inflammation and autism—was presented in the 1998 article in "The Lancet" as an interpretation and not a definite association, but in the articles

(Wakefield 2003) and in the many interviews that followed, he abandoned this caution, forcefully maintaining the causal relationship. It was not the first time that Wakefield toyed with fanciful associations, but to fully understand the plan he had in mind, we have to take a step back in time.

Five years earlier, he had already aroused amazement in the scientific community when he had hypothesized a nexus between a chronic inflammatory disease of the intestine, known as Crohn's disease, and the measles virus (Wakefield et al. 1993). Two years later, again in "The Lancet", he added a nexus with the vaccine for measles (Thompson et al. 1995). Concerned by these dubious theories, in 1998 the chief medical inspector of the British Ministry of Health, together with a group of experts, analysed the research, concluding that there were no data to support an association between Crohn's disease, measles and the anti-measles vaccine. Wakefield thus decided to drop the accusation against this acute form of intestinal inflammation, but only to hone his weapons and prepare a more appealing and profitable hypothesis. In the same period, he filed a number of patents: in 1995, one for a method to diagnose Crohn's colitis and ulcerative colitis through the presence in the intestine of the virus of measles—moreover, using not the address of the research institute, according to practice, but his private home address—and in 1997 (8 months before the scientific article) the patent for a "safer" anti-measles vaccine, namely a monodose vaccine that should have replaced the combined trivalent one then available, considered more dangerous because it contained the two viruses of mumps and rubella, which were capable, according to Wakefield, of triggering off intestinal inflammation and therefore autism (Deer 2011b). The plan consisted of throwing discredit on the trivalent vaccination, accusing it of causing autism, in order to then put his own rival product on the market: a vaccine with a single dose of measles. A few days before the publication of the article, Wakefield held a press conference to publicize the results of his research, suggested parents demand monodose vaccines for their children and distributed a convincing video in which some alarmed families accused the vaccines (Deer 2011a): this type of behaviour was totally atypical for a scientist and, as we will see (in Chap. 4) is usually that of quacks. In addition, from as early as 1996, Wakefield had started to work with a lawyer, Richard Barr of the Dawnbarns law firm, who was attempting a class action against the companies manufacturing trivalent vaccines. The collaboration had also taken place through the medical-legal consulting firm of Carmel O'Donovan Associates—managed by Wakefield's wife, Carmel O'Donovan, before the scandal broke out—, which issued the invoices relative to Wakefield's consulting work. The compromise of Wakefield went even further: some of the 12 children "selected" for his experiment came from families belonging to the anti-vaccination group JABS (Justice, Awareness & Basic Support: The Support Group for Vaccine Damaged Children), which was preparing for compensation lawsuits for the damage caused by vaccinations thanks to the legal help of Barr—who had filed a claim for damages (with money from the Legal Aid Board, the government fund for people who cannot afford legal assistance) which became a cheque for £55,000 to the hospital and £435,643 for Wakefield (paid to the company in his wife's name) with the aim of funding his research. This was an abnormal conflict of interest which had to be made known and which it was compulsory to state in scientific publications. If the strategic scheme had gone as planned, the Wakefield monodose vaccine would have replaced the trivalent vaccine in England, and perhaps elsewhere, with a considerable economic return (the tabloid "The Sun" estimated it at around £38 million per year).

Let's go back to 1998. As soon as the article was published in "The Lancet", the scientific community expressed its doubts on Wakefield's conclusions. However it took them seriously, deeming them wrong but genuine. In the following months and years, various articles were published which, starting from wider samples of the population, reached different conclusions, not being able to find any connection between the trivalent vaccine, intestinal inflammation and autism. In the meantime, the social psychosis for the trivalent MMR grew out of all proportion, and the herd immunity of the British population dropped dangerously under the safety threshold, reaching, in the 2-year period 2003/04, 79.9%. The climate of discredit towards the trivalent vaccination lasted for no less than 6 years (until 2004), during which Wakefield proved that he was an excellent communicator: in interviews and on TV programmes he was skilfully able to involve the then Prime Minister Tony Blair declaring (which was not true) that even his youngest son had not received the trivalent vaccine; in November 2000, he organized a tour of lectures in the United States and appeared in a long television programme on the CBS channel, stating that the trivalent was linked to the "current epidemic of autism". In a few months, the ranks of the American anti-vaccine movements swelled. In the end, it was a journalist from the "Sunday Times" who revealed that it was all a fraud: Brian Deer,[8] thanks to a meticulous and long investigation which lasted 7 years, from 2003 to 2011, but made public from February 2004 (Deer 2004). As well as the conflict of interest, Deer

---

[8] This and much other information is not the opinions of the writer but documented facts. The documents that prove unequivocally the fraudulent attitude of Wakefield—which after in-depth confirmations led to the British health institutions deciding to strike the doctor off the Medical Register—are public and can be consulted by anyone on the site of the "Sunday Times" journalist, Brian Deer, http://tinyurl.com/yao23ye

checked the data collected by Wakefield and interviewed the twelve families of children chosen as the sample: the plan of a "deliberate fraud" thus emerged (Deer 2011a, b; Godlee et al. 2011). In the first place Deer realized that the sample had been deliberately created to prove the harmfulness of the vaccine, i.e. that the twelve children had been chosen not randomly from the small patients of the Royal Free Hospital in London (as stated in the article) but recruited from anti-vaccination families with children suffering from cognitive disabilities—none of the patients came from London and one had even been recruited in the United States. In the second place, Wakefield falsified the clinical records and manipulated the data: some of the children had shown characteristics of autism *before* being given the vaccine, whereas others were not affected at all by autism. In the third place, Wakefield had subjected the disabled children to invasive and superfluous diagnostic examinations, such as a colonoscopy and lumbar punctures, without the parents' consent.

In March 2004, after these investigations had been made public, 10 out of the 12 co-authors of Wakefield's article sent a note retracting their conclusions to "The Lancet" (Murch et al. 2004). In the same issue there appeared a long note by the editor of the journal, Richard Horton, who listed the hypothesis of scientific misconduct in six points. In the light of the accusations and the documents collected by Deer, the British General Medical Council (GMC) opened an investigation to examine the data of Wakefield reaching, in January 2010, a verdict that the accusations were fully grounded: 4 episodes of dishonesty and manipulation of scientific data and one of abuse of disabled children. In February the same year, 12 years after the publication, "The Lancet" retracted the article with an unsigned editorial, a sign that it was expressing the unanimous opinion of the editors. On the basis of the conclusions of the GMC, which considered Wakefield "dishonest, immoral and insensitive", especially to young disabled patients, in May 2010, the Council struck him off the Medical Register, banning him from exercising the medical profession in the United Kingdom. Wakefield then moved to the United States, where he still continues to profess his "theories".

Perhaps due to the long duration—6 years were necessary before any doubts emerged in the newspapers and twelve before the article was retracted by the scientific journal—the effects of this scientific fraud were devastating. Before going on to examine them, it is interesting to note how the very many attempts by the scientific community to prove the inconsistency of Wakefield's thesis were of little use. The figures are impressive: between the year of publication of the article, 1998, and 2014, 107 articles were published, which from various points of view proved how there was no relation between the trivalent MMR vaccine and autism, but only a meaningless casual temporal coincidence. It is instructive to see the conclusions of some of these studies, to see first-hand the extent to which irrationality and the emotiveness of decision-making choices of some parents can be driven.

Probably in order to balance the lightness with which it had assessed Wakefield's article, "The Lancet" was the first to publish in the following 2 years two extensive longitudinal works (including an extensive prospective study, where a *longitudinal prospective study* consists of following in time two groups of individuals, one exposed and the other not, to a presumed cause of disease, in order to compare their respective risks), focused on large populations (three million individuals) belonging to the age group subject to the trivalent vaccine, from which it emerged that statistically the onset of autism, gastrointestinal disorders and administration of the vaccine are three phenomena which are not correlated (Peltola et al. 1998; Taylor et al. 1999). It was then proven that the time window in which the three events appeared in the patients is very wide, and in any case without any cause-effect relationship (DeStefano and Thompson 2004; Afzal et al. 2006; Hornig et al. 2008). Every year, since 1998, on average two or three epidemiological studies are published, produced by independent researchers, who stress the lack of causality between the trivalent vaccine and autism, and in the past few years, also thanks to the availability of programs that can manage enormous amounts of data—the so-called *big data*—studies are published which weigh up the data from several millions of vaccinated children and data banks (Vaccine Safety Datalink) for any adverse reactions (McNeil et al. 2014) and which prove how world epidemiology exonerates the trivalent vaccine from any responsibility whatsoever in the onset of manifestations of the autistic spectrum (Roehr 2013; DeStefano et al. 2013; Gentile et al. 2013; Deisher et al. 2015).

As time has passed, the studies have concentrated on the years and the countries in which the trivalent vaccine has been introduced or eliminated from the vaccinal calendar, to understand whether it was possible to observe increases or decreases of the rate of autism in the population. According to expectations, the administration of the trivalent has not had an impact on the increasing trend of the cases of autism and, above all, this pathology is not more common in children who have been vaccinated with respect to those who have not—in the case examined by Madsen, the sample is represented by all Danish children, half a million, born between 1991 and 1998 (Dales et al. 2001; Madsen et al. 2002). Other works have compared a population of autistic subjects and one of healthy subjects, used as a control sample, proving that they received the trivalent vaccine at the same time and quantity (Uno et al. 2015), and that not even between autistic and normal siblings (therefore in families with a strong predisposition) an identical vaccinal calendar causes autism (Jain et al. 2015). One study in particular has proven that the increase in the rate of autism in the British population has undergone neither variations in the period of the introduction of the trivalent vaccine nor stabilizations, even though the rate of trivalent vaccination is constant (Kaye et al. 2001). Some studies have directly observed the effects of the agents accused of stimulating the onset of autism, for example evaluating the presence of the antibodies of measles (sign of a past infection or vaccination) in autistic and normal children, without finding differences in the two groups (D'Souza et al. 2006; Baird et al. 2008), or inoculating in macaques different doses of trivalent vaccine containing the dreaded preservative ethylmercury without obtaining any harmful effect (Gadad et al. 2015). Lastly, scientific literature is practically unanimous in attributing the rate of autism not to a real growth of this disorder but to an increase and refinement in the diagnostic criteria, as behaviour which today is categorized as belonging to the autistic spectrum was excluded up to about 10 years ago (Hansen et al. 2015; Jick et al. 2003; Merrick et al. 2004; Taylor 2006; Nassar et al. 2009; Blumberg et al. 2013).

These studies collect a huge amount of impressive data which leaves no doubt at all on their validity: they summarize the analyses of tens of millions of individuals of varying ages and with different genetics, made by hundreds of independent researchers from different public research centres in various countries. Any criticisms of preference or referred to conflicts of interest are, therefore, inadmissible and meaningless. Yet, all these results were not able to stem a scientific fraud conducted on 12 children. As mentioned, those who are profoundly convinced that vaccines cause autism do not change their minds even if brought face to face with these self-evident results and not even in the face of the most incontestable evidence: the rate of autism has increased in a population even though the trivalent vaccine has been suspended! This evidence exists and was shown by a Japanese study in 2005. It is interesting to summarize this study for its simplicity and clarity which make it accessible to a public of non-experts (Honda et al. 2005).

Japan, after having introduced it in 1989, is the only country to have suspended the trivalent vaccination in 1993, opting for monovalent doses of measles, mumps and rubella: it, therefore, represents a fortuitous natural experiment to test any trivalent-autism relationship. The study was conducted on a population of 300,000 children born in the Yokohama area between 1988 and 1996 and continued for 7 years. In this period of time, 278 cases of autistic spectrum disorders (ASD), 158 cases of autism and 120 cases of minor autistic conditions were diagnosed; of the cases of autism, 60 showed a certain regression during development (losing skills already acquired) and 12 a probable regression. In the group born in 1988, 70% of the children had been

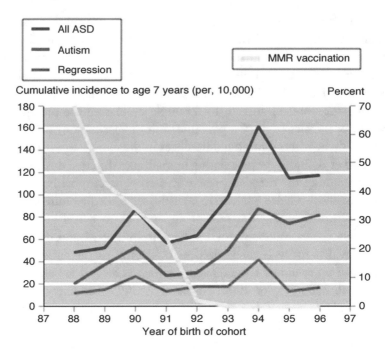

**Fig. 3.1** MMR vaccination rates by year of birth (1988–1992) in the city of Yokohama, annual trends of cumulative incidence of autistic spectrum disorders (ASD), with and without developmental regression, up to 7 years of age, in the birth cohort object of the study (image by Bandolier 2005, redrawn after Honda et al. 2005)

vaccinated with the trivalent, in 1992 only 1.8% and from 1993 the percentage goes to 0, as the trivalent had been taken off the market. As the diagram in the following figure shows, the rate of autism and autistic spectrum disorders continues to grow despite the suspension of the trivalent vaccine. It can be noted that autism begins to grow with children born from 1992 onwards, i.e. those who had not been vaccinated and is less in children born before 1992, to whom the vaccine had been administered. It is difficult to imagine how such evidence can be rejected, yet it is (Fig. 3.1).

Not only have these studies been unable to demolish the false relationship between autism and the trivalent vaccine, but they have not even stemmed a widespread discredit of other vaccinations and the following decline in herd immunity, with effects which in the United Kingdom have been fatal. Wakefield's media campaign has, unfortunately, had a wide impact on the population, undermining the trust in vaccinations of some generations of young parents (Poland and Spier 2010). In the 6 years previous to 1998 in England, the rate of trivalent MMR vaccination oscillated around 92%, but after the 1998 media campaign, it started to drop, and in the 2 years 2003/ 2004 it reached its lowest point, 79.9%, which means that in that year 100,000 children were not vaccinated. It was only from 2005 onwards that the cover of the population slowly began to grow again, but still without having reached the threshold of 95%, recommended by the WHO as safe.

The consequences were not long in coming: between 2008 and 2009, for the first time in 14 years, measles was once again declared endemic in England and Wales with 2500 cases (in 2010 there had been 380). However, the epidemic did not explode until 2012, with almost 10,000 cases of mumps which caused the death of 14 babies under 3 months and the simultaneous epidemic of measles which between 2012 and 2013 recorded 3303 cases, of which 257 were admitted to hospital, 39 severe cases of encephalitis, meningitis, pneumonia and gastroenteritis, the death of a child plus two other deaths in the following 2 years.[9] To understand the direct responsibilities of this pandemic and deaths, we have to observe the age groups most attacked by measles.[10] Figures 3.2 and 3.3 analyse the population of two large British regions in 2012 and 2013 and show that the age group which recorded the greatest number of cases of measles and which has least vaccinal cover is that of adolescents (10–15 years old) or the children of parents influenced by the media campaign originated by Wakefield's fraud (Tannous et al. 2014; Calvert et al. 2013; Battistella et al. 2013; Brown et al. 2012; Bates 2011; Poland and Spier 2010).

This is the dramatic and glaring proof of how false research, relaunched by the Internet non-critically, can become a tangible danger for the whole community; it is a danger which, in all probability, has not yet been defeated. To be effective, the trivalent MMR vaccine needs a second administration, known as a booster dose, around the age of five or six, as the epidemic of mumps which between 2002 and 2006 affected the United States, the Netherlands and England shows (in the last case reaching 56,000 infections in 2005 alone), mainly affecting the age group of between 18 and 24—the majority of which (between 70 and 88%) discovered because immunized with a single dose of trivalent (Kutty et al. 2010; Roggendorf et al. 2010). The Wakefield affair has already influenced the generation of children born in the years

---

[9] Oxford Vaccine group, Vaccine Knowledge Project, Measles, http://tinyurl.com/jlktxgc; Public Health England. The National Archives, Mumps Notifications in England and Wales by Age Group, 1989–2012, http://tinyurl.com/2ug45bb; Public Health England, Infection report/Immunisation, Vol. 9, N. 42, 27 November 2015, http://tinyurl.com/jb2gqte; Public Health England, Measles Deaths by Age Group: 1980–2013, http://tinyurl.com/l4soqef

[10] Public Health England, The National Archives, Confirmed Cases of Measles by Region and Age: 1996–2013, http://tinyurl.com/2ug45bb

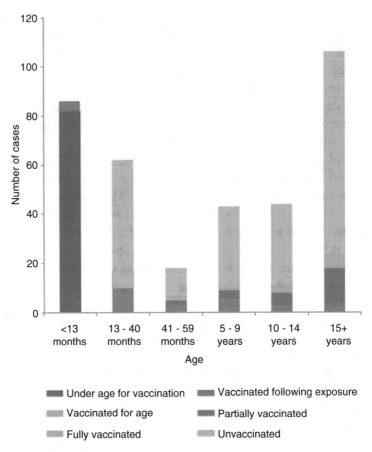

**Fig. 3.2** Vaccinal cover of the trivalent measles–mumps–rubella vaccine by age, confirmed cases of measles (*n* = 359), Merseyside (pop. 1.4 million), UK, January–June 2012 (redrawn after Vivancos et al. 2012)

immediately following 1998, who avoided the first administration but it is probable that it can also act on the older generations who in those years should have had the booster injection but avoided it. Future epidemiological analyses will reveal whether they are also to be counted among the victims of Wakefield (Godlee et al. 2011).

The case of autism is not the only one of discredit against vaccines based on falsified or omitted data. Another case, very widespread on the Internet, maintains that "scientists are divided" on the issue of the safety of vaccinations, suggesting that it is a "scientifically controversial procedure". It is absolutely not true that scientists are divided, let alone that the safety of vaccines is a controversial topic. We have to look at the figures and the evidence here as well.

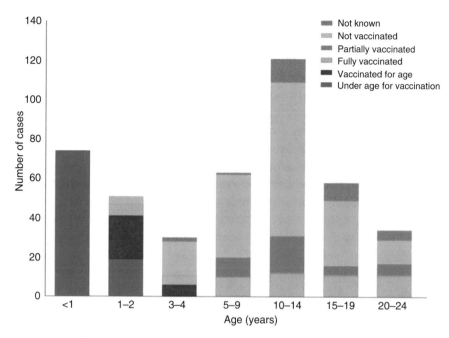

**Fig. 3.3** Vaccinal cover of the trivalent measles–mumps–rubella vaccine by age, confirmed and probable cases of measles ($n = 486$), Greater Manchester (pop. 2.7 million), UK, Otcober 2012–September 2013 (redrawn after Pegorie et al. 2014)

A census of 2014 established that the number of doctors active in the United States was equal to 916,264, with notoriously anti-vaccination doctors numbering about 200, i.e. 0.02% of the total, an extremely small minority (but who make a lot of noise in the media) comparable with that of other Western countries (Young et al. 2015).[11] Criticisms have also emerged in Italy on vaccinations from that minority of medical circles which join the anti-vaccination parents. In October 2015, several newspapers published an open letter signed by 120 doctors addressed to the President of the Istituto Superiore di Sanità (equivalent to the US NIH), in which they expressed a series of doubts on the quantity and procedures of vaccinations. The letter, skilfully,

---

[11] The approximate average of 200 units emerges from an analysis of the following four lists: the first one, the only one which calculates the number of only doctors (with some exceptions) lists 52 anti-vaccinationist doctors, the second and third lists which add in the list doctors and scientists with a Ph.D. list, respectively, 81 and 279 scientists contrary to or critical of vaccinations. The last list brings together some 300 doctors who have a friendly approach to vaccinations—many of the same names appear in the different lists. (1) Sceptical Raptor—Stalking pseudoscience in the internet jungle. Anti-vaccine doctors—naming names and listing lists, 2017/06/18: https://goo.gl/gGmjh3; (2) The Vienna Report: https://goo.gl/iXyzG1; (3) Malaysian Vaccines Exposed: https://goo.gl/eHJVwk (4) Best Vaccine Friendly Doctor List: https://goo.gl/zkd9sr

did not state that it was simply against vaccinations and actually began with the following statement: "Today, any doctor with common sense and a minimum of scientific knowledge cannot be against paediatric vaccinations and we all know the utility of this health practice". Those who study anti-vaccination movements know the rhetorical strategy very well, typical, in general of the most radical anti-vaccinationists, and which has them begin by saying: "I am not an anti-vaccinationist, but …". This deceitful artifice is similar to the typical racist who before listing a series of accusations against minorities, begins with: "I am not a racist but …"; when someone starts this way, you can be fairly sure that you have a stalwart anti-vaccinationist in front of you. After this statement of principle (only), in the body of the letter a series of general fears are raised—never supported by data, evidence or scientific articles, but shown with rhetorical and scientifically irrelevant expressions such as "it is known that" and "parents tell us", aimed at maintaining that vaccinated children are immunologically weaker and therefore more exposed to diseases than those who are not vaccinated, focusing attention on the presumed excessive antigenic load of multiple vaccines and on the toxic components of the adjuvants and preservatives. We will return in the next chapter to the scientific inconsistency of these theories, without the minimum requirements of the experimental method and other similar attempts to delegitimize vaccines from a pseudo-scientific point of view. For the time being, it is significant here to examine only the numerical aspect, as it is the most recurrent in the false argument of "science is divided".

A parent who reads an appeal by 120 doctors expressing doubts about vaccination could effectively be worried. We have to reflect on the fact that as science is a free activity without dogmas, it does not require 100% adhesion by experts to declare a theory or a therapy valid and effective. In all disciplinary fields, 100% acceptance exists on hardly any fact or theory—for example, in biology, there is always a small group of heretics who oppose Darwin's theory of natural selection, for reasons that are either ideological or religious, even though it has been supported by a mass of incontrovertible data. The same applied to the causal relationship between infection by the HIV virus and the onset of AIDS: it has been widely shown, but now and again, there are some outlandish doctors around the world who deny this evidence (possibly to sell alternative homotoxicological products or antiviral therapies).

The same, naturally, applies to vaccines. However, as in the American case, looking at the numbers, the problem disappears. One hundred and twenty doctors signed the appeal, while the other 350,000, or the remainder of doctors in Italy, do not express any doubts: the real ratio is, therefore, 99.7% of doctors in favour against 0.03% who express "doubts". Science is not divided at all, as can be seen, and the numbers supporting this imaginary division are false, lacking or partially perceived. That 0.03% appears more numerous because it makes a loud noise in the media: the "dissidents" of medicine play the media role of victims excluded from the system; they give interviews and appear on TV but they are careful from arguing their theories in scientific journals to which they could send detailed studies corroborated by incontrovertible data, to prove their theories and earn lasting fame. This is never the case, obviously. I will leave it to the reader to guess why.

Apart from the topic of "heavy metals" already discussed, there is another subject focused on the chemical compounds in which the data are manipulated to instil fear about vaccinations: the supposed toxicity of the excipients. To deal with this, we could simply refer to the vast documentation produced by the two main Western agencies for the safety of drugs, the US FDA[12] and the European Medicines Agency (EMA),[13] which with special procedures certify the thresholds of toxicity of all drugs, including the various excipients used to preserve, stabilize and boost the vaccines. Even though the radical anti-vaccinationists refuse this subject, it is worthwhile remembering that these regulatory agencies (as will be explained in detail in Chap. 5) are independent international bodies, and that each country has its regulatory agency, with its own procedures of verification and collection of any adverse effects. Even if there were to be cases of corruption or conflicts of interest, their number and the transparency of their data—which can be checked by anyone on their respective websites—makes it unthinkable that they could be subjected to any economic or political influence. However, beyond these arguments of common sense and solid documentary evidence produced by the international agencies, let's look at the proof that demolishes the most frequent accusations of toxicity, using two essential concepts to understand the nature of any pharmacological treatment: doses and times of administration. Let's start, as always, from history.

As early as the origins of pharmacological thought, the Swiss doctor and alchemist Paracelsus (1493–1541) maintained in 1538: "Everything is poison, nothing exists that is not poisonous; only the dose means that the poison has no effect". Even earlier than him, in classical Greece, in the Hellenistic period, medical thought had questioned the use of natural substances for therapeutic purposes, with the compilation of recipe books, lists of antidotes and herbalists which began to list the therapeutic or toxic virtues of plants, animals and

---

[12] FDA, Vaccines, Blood & Biologics, Safety & Availability, Vaccine Safety & Availability, Common Ingredients in U.S. Licensed Vaccines, http://tinyurl.com/q8djboh
[13] EMA, Guideline on Adjuvants in Vaccines for Human Use, http://tinyurl.com/z3fuyvj

minerals, thus defining the concept of *pharmakon*, a preparation which each time could be a curative product, a poison or a drug (Conforti et al. 2012, p. 88). Modern pharmacology fully confirms these ancient intuitions—and the contrary occurs even more often, i.e. that it is modern science that proves the naivety or the errors of the past; in both cases, however, history remains a very instructive tool. We have already mentioned water, the commonest element swallowed everyday by man, which can become toxic or even fatal if taken in large quantities after stress. Meat is also recommended in diets, but an excess of meat, especially processed (frankfurters), if prolonged for some decades, may have carcinogenic effects, as has recently been reported—without due dissemination skill—by the IARC, the international agency for research on cancer. The same applies for the effective and common aspirin which, as mentioned, can become toxic if the times and doses of administration are not respected. The reasoning can be reversed from innocuous to poisonous molecules. The botulin toxin is produced by the bacteria, harmless in itself, *Clostridium botulinum*, and it is one of the most fatal poisons known—it only takes 0.00000003 milligrams of botulin A toxin per kilogram of body weight to kill an individual—and it is, to give an example, a million times more powerful than the dreaded dioxin, a powerful poison synthesized chemically by man; yet, small amounts of the purified toxin, capable of interrupting the nervous impulses and induce muscular paralysis, can become an efficient treatment for diseases with uncontrolled spasms (in particular those of the eyelids and of the bladder) and it is also used in cosmetics, under the commercial name of Botox, to temporarily smooth out wrinkles (Le Couteur and Burreson 2006, p. 56; Silvestrini 2014, p. 12; Vozza et al. 2017, p. 62). The examples could continue, from antibiotics to lifesaving antitumour drugs: everything depends on the dose and time of exposure of the organism. These are fundamental concepts for pharmacology, and in order to understand them specific competences are necessary. They also imply the notion of risk: a mixture that is explosive for navigators of the Internet, who come across the descriptions of the composition of the drugs and excipients of the vaccines, alarming themselves and others.

As far as the case of vaccines is concerned, naturally there is nothing toxic in them and it is hard to understand why there should be. All the molecules in them are well known, listed in explanatory leaflets and on the websites of the regulatory agencies. Their safety emerges from the epidemiological data, monitored every week by the WHO, coming from millions of vaccinated individuals all over the world. The excipients added to the vials essentially carry out three important functions: they preserve, stabilize and boost the content of the vaccines. Let's start from the preservatives, used to keep the vials sterile, preventing the formation of infectious agents. They include thiomersal and formaldehyde, greatly criticized by the Internet. Thiomersal is one of the most obvious cases of the irrationality of the fears of vaccines and closely recalls the Japanese case of the suspension of the trivalent vaccine: its elimination, very similar to what happened in Yokohama, has not caused in the population a decrease in the neurological and immunity diseases of which it was accused. The relative diagrams in scientific literature show how, while decreasing the line of distribution of thiomersal in the North American population since 1999, the line of the rate of neurotoxic pathologies not only does not fall but over the years tends to increase[14] (Madsen et al. 2003; Verstraeten et al. 2003; Montana et al. 2010; Baggs et al. 2011). In this case too, there have been no public amends by those who causally correlated neurological diseases with paediatric vaccines based on thiomersal; on the contrary, many websites still online and some "B" rate scientific publications continue to hypothesize possible risks.

The fear of formaldehyde is also unjustified and based on data reported incorrectly. Formaldehyde is a component which is used at low concentrations to fix the cells in the different phases of laboratory experiments and at high concentrations (as in the case of formalin) to preserve biological tissues; it is found in the liquid state in the typical cylindrical containers of anatomical museums to preserve biological exhibits. It is a powerful bactericide, because it prevents the protein bonds that allow infectious agents to replicate, and formaldehyde is actually used in producing vaccines to obtain the toxoids, i.e. toxins produced by pathogens (as in the case of tetanus and diphtheria) which with formaldehyde lose their toxicity while keeping their ability to activate the immune system and to produce vaccines based on microorganisms that have been killed (not based on attenuated living microorganisms, like the Sabin oral anti-polio vaccine or the vaccine for tuberculosis). At high concentrations, formaldehyde is carcinogenic, as are very many substances; the prolonged consumption of alcohol is certainly carcinogenic as is prolonged exposure to the sun; there is a good probability that the smoke from fried food is also carcinogenic, as is the daily and unprotected contact with products for hair colouring, sawdust from hard woods (e.g. *Mansonia altissima*) and 20 cups of coffee a day for decades.[15] The dose of formaldehyde present in vaccines is absolutely not carcinogenic and for at least three reasons. First of all,

---

[14] Danish Study Does Not Support Hypothesis of Association Between Thiomersal and Autism, "Eurosurveillance", Vol. 7, N. 41, 9 October 2003.

[15] International Agency for Research on Cancer, Agents Classified by the IARC Monographs, Volumes 1–112: http://tinyurl.com/nedj8qf

formaldehyde is one of the essential intermediaries of the human metabolism necessary for the synthesis of the basic constituents both of the proteins and of the nucleic acids (the nitrogen bases) which form the support for the genetic material (purines and pyrimidines). For this reason, formaldehyde is regularly present in our blood circulation in a concentration of about 2.5 µg for every millilitre of blood. Toxicological research has shown that in a child of 2 months weighing about 5 kg, with an average quantity of blood equal to 85 ml per kilogram, the total amount of formaldehyde produced naturally present in the blood circulation is approximately equal to 1.1 mg: 10 times greater than that contained in the vaccines. In the second place, animal tests show that not even vaccines that contain 600 times the dose of formaldehyde present in human vaccines show signs of toxicity (Natarajan et al. 1983; Til et al. 1989; Offit and Jew 2003; Heck and Casanova 2004). Lastly, doses of formaldehyde greater than those in vaccines are taken almost every day in the diet, either because it is artificially present in the preservatives (E-240) of many foods, especially tinned fish, or because it is naturally present in tomatoes, potatoes, pears, apples, carrots, watermelons, apricots, bananas and cauliflower.[16]

Another important category of excipients are the adjuvants. These are substances which stimulate some cells of the immune system to improve the efficacy of the vaccine and the duration of its memory, also reducing the number of immunologically active molecules (antigens) capable of activating the production of antibodies. The derivatives of alum, monophosphoryl lipid A and oil emulsions, belong to adjuvants. Aluminium salts, of which the safety profiles are well known, have been used for about 70 years in the field of vaccines and are used, for example, in the trivalent anti-diphtheria–anti-tetanus–anti-pertussis (acellular) vaccine, the pneumococcal conjugate vaccine and the vaccine against hepatitis B. The two prime suspects in this category are squalene and aluminium. Squalene is a biological substance that is very important for the life of organisms, because it is involved in the construction of steroid hormones and other lipidic substances, as well as in the synthesis of cholesterol (of which it fights the harmful effects) which takes place in the liver. It is found in the sebum of human skin and is present in very many plants and animals, including the shark (where its name comes from) which is rich in it because being less dense than water it contributes to its hydrostatic thrust, supporting its considerable mass. Squalene is also present in eggs, in olive oil and sometimes, artificially, in cosmetics like mascara, lipstick and talcum powder; it is also used in vaccines because, as well as being easily extractable,

---

[16] European Food Safety Authority, Endogenous Formaldehyde Turnover in Humans Compared with Exogenous Contribution from Food Sources, "EFSA Journal", 2014, 12(2), p. 3550.

it has proven to be an excellent stimulant of the immune response. As squalene is a product of synthesis of our body and having gone through all the control procedures, it is considered completely safe and therefore has been administered to several million people, and it has never produced any unwanted effects. For several years, however, websites, blogs and word of mouth have considered it (perhaps only because of the sinister name) a suspect for the presumed neurological damage caused by vaccines, even though, for the reasons mentioned above, the problem of the harmfulness of the dose or the costs/benefits balance cannot even be raised. The fear of squalene is, in short, a meaningless "meme", one of the many ideas that are spread by pure emulation through the Internet and which, becoming famous, gain the status of truth even when this is completely unfounded.

The case of alum is different, because it entails the notion of toxicity. The website accuses the derivatives of aluminium present in the vaccines, deeming them capable of inducing neurotoxicity and fostering the onset of Alzheimer's disease and breast cancer. These last two examples are to be rejected because the negative outcomes of the experimental tests have cleared alum (Lidsky 2014; Namer et al. 2008). The question of neurotoxicity is real but, once again, it is linked to times and doses of exposure (altered by the Internet): although the regulatory bodies were fully aware of the maximum doses not to be exceeded as adjuvants; over the years different studies have been carried out to see whether the accumulation of aluminium in the diet of children[17] and in the different vaccines present in the vaccinal calendar (0–36 months) came within the threshold called *minimum level of risk*.[18] It emerged that, in the first year of life (that of greatest sensitivity), babies receive a quantity of aluminium from vaccines and food that is "significantly below" the safe doses—and therefore, continuing to use paediatric vaccines that contain aluminium represents an "extremely low risk" which "exceeds any theoretical concern" (Keith et al. 2002; Mitkus et al. 2011). The vaccines also contain stabilizers (albumen, glycine, phenols and monosodium glutamate), suspension fluids (saline solution, sterile water) and in some cases antibiotics (not penicillin) to avoid the development of germs, a growth medium for viruses or bacteria (mainly proteins from hen's eggs in doses and conditions such as to avoid, with rare exceptions, reactions in people who are allergic) and some carbohydrates such as glucides, to trigger the immune response (this is the case of the conjugate

---

[17] Safety of Aluminium from Dietary Intake, Dietary Exposure to Aluminium-Containing Food Additives 2013 (Question Number: Efsa-Q-2013-00312), "EFSA Journal", 2008, 754, pp. 1–34.

[18] The Agency for Toxic Substances and Disease Registry, Aluminum (CAS ID #: 7429-90-5), http://tinyurl.com/zdjvfto

vaccines against pneumococcus and meningococcus, covered with polysaccharides): there are minor criticisms of these compounds (Offit and Jew 2003), which have not reached the popularity of the cases mentioned above. However, it cannot be ruled out that in the future this may come about: fashions and the fears of the Internet have rules that are not always comprehensible.

There are two more subjects worthy of note regarding the manipulation of data. The first concerns the vaccinal overload, the other the inefficacy of vaccines in reducing historical infections. In the previous chapter, we already in part mentioned the topic of vaccinal overload regarding soldiers and children, observing how solid scientific literature proves that the professional categories most vaccinated do not show a weakened immune system, or a greater rate of tumours, and that during seasonal infections, children are subjected to a natural immune stimulation that is dozens of times greater than the artificial ones caused by vaccines. More recently, however, the spread of fears by parents has encouraged new research to look more closely at this topic. In the next chapter, we will again return to the hypothesis of vaccinal overload observing how, compared to non-vaccinated children, those vaccinated against measles have a better resistance to infectious diseases and live longer. It is now worth approaching the problem in more general terms, quoting the results of two recent interesting experiments. The first examined a sample of over 1000 American children, of 7, 12 and 24 months of age, measuring how their immune system was stimulated by the different vaccines through the antigenic load, to evaluate possible neurophysiological effects during the different phases of development monitored up to 7–10 years of age. The result showed that the lesser or greater vaccinal stimulation in the first 2 years of life has no effect on the neurocognitive development of the children (Iqbal et al. 2013). The second experiment, on the other hand, directly tackled the topic of the weakening of the immune system, comparing its reactivity to diseases in two groups of children, one vaccinated and the other not, for a total of over 13,000 children and adolescents between the ages of 1 and 17. The study, therefore, measured the respective prevalence of three categories of diseases: the infectious ones preventable by vaccinations (mumps, measles, rubella, whooping cough), those that are not preventable by vaccinations (flu, tonsillitis, infection from herpes virus, bronchitis, gastrointestinal infections, cystitis and/or urethritis, purulent bacterial conjunctivitis, laryngotracheitis) and some general and allergic diseases (allergic rhinoconjunctivitis, eczema, bronchial asthma, obstructive bronchitis, pneumonia and otitis media, heart diseases, anaemia, epilepsy, attention deficit disorder/hyperactivity). The result was twofold. In the first place, the group that had not been vaccinated had a much higher rate of measles, whooping cough and mumps compared to the vaccinated group—rubella gave a statistically insignificant result—showing that they were more at risk of infection from severe or fatal diseases. On the other hand, as far as the other two types of diseases are concerned, i.e. those which cannot be prevented by vaccinations and the miscellaneous and allergic ones, the two groups did not show significant statistical variations: both fell ill with the same frequency, proving that the immune system of those who receive multiple vaccinations is not weakened at all. However, considering that the two groups are level for two categories of diseases but not for the first one (infectious diseases preventable with vaccinations), their sum shows that the vaccinated children, falling ill much less with pertussis, measles and mumps in the first 10 years of life, overall enjoy better health (Schmitz et al. 2011). It has to be specified that this study resumes and confirms two other vast epidemiological studies on the supposed relations between vaccinations and allergies: in one it was proven that the children who had received the vaccination for *Haemophilus influenzae* and the two trivalent diphtheria–tetanus–pertussis (DTP) and for measles–mumps–rubella (MMR) had not developed a greater allergic sensitivity compared to the population (Bernsen et al. 2006); in the other, which involved more than 2000 children aged between the age of 1 and 2, it was proven that the effect of the vaccination in the first year of life did not increase the allergic sensitivity and atopic dermatitis in the second year of life (Gruber et al. 2008).

One last reflection regarding the manipulation of data must be dedicated to the various fanciful reconstructions in circulation on the Internet which tend to deny or reduce the effects of vaccinations in eradicating infectious diseases and in the increase in the life expectancy in the twentieth century. These reconstructions are not truthful for two orders of reasons. In the first place, in the vast majority of cases, misleading diagrams are shown, from which it would emerge how infectious diseases drop not in correspondence with the introduction of the vaccines, but before or after them—attributing the responsibility for the drop not to the vaccines but to the improvement in hygiene and health conditions. The data in these diagrams are often falsified or fabricated; however, even when there is no manipulation, the way they are shown is deceitful and tends to confuse the reader. It is a fairly refined way to deliver frauds in science and it is more difficult to identify—perhaps for this reason it is worthy of little attention by the debunkers. Let's take the case of whooping cough. On the Internet, there are many diagrams that show how, well before the introduction of the trivalent tetanus–diphtheria–pertussis to the United States in 1948, whooping cough had already been strongly declining for at least 20 years, a sign that would induce the surfer of the web to consider the vaccine useless. In this case, however, one invalidating fact is omitted, namely that the vaccine for pertussis alone (and not combined with others in the trivalent vaccines) was introduced in 1914 (Baker and Katz 2004) playing a significant role, but omitted from the diagrams, in the drop in pertussis in the years preceding 1948. Another typical case consists of choosing to represent, depending on the cases, the "mortality rate" (the ratio between the average population in a given period of time and the number of deaths in a community) or the "disease rate" (the proportion between new infectious events and the population in which they occur, in a given period of time), using windows of time and units of measurement in a misleading way. In the case of diphtheria, for example, diagrams circulate on the Internet which show how in a limited period of time the spread of the vaccine for diphtheria (in particular in 1926 as an antiserum and in 1947/48 as a combined vaccination with anti-tetanus) did not decrease in the immediate period the rate of mortality. In this case, it is clear that thousands of people with diphtheria continued to die even after the introduction of the vaccine, as it was a preventive procedure—a prophylaxis—which takes several months to spread and become efficient. If, on the other hand, the index of the spread of the disease in a correct period of time is used (one decade before and one after suffice), an immediate collapse in the cases of the spread and rate of the disease can be clearly observed, when the vaccine arrives on the market.

Similar manipulations also apply for smallpox, typhoid fever, scarlet fever and other infective diseases. This does not mean, of course, that the better hygiene and socio-economic conditions did not contribute to eradicating the infectious diseases preventable by vaccinations. Better hospitals, the development of pharmacological, surgical and clinical-diagnostic knowledge, the implementation of institutions to foster public health and the spread of health and hygiene practices for the population—and that in the twentieth century the illiteracy rate fell from 56% to 1.5%—played their role in limiting the spread and the health effects of infectious diseases; but not to consider the vaccines as principally responsible for this collective well-being is to turn reality upside-down.

In the second place, to evaluate the falsity of these reconstructions of the recent past, exemplary cases are offered by modernity, where significant variations in the hygienic and cultural conditions can certainly not be called into question. In 1989, when the Soviet Union collapsed, the crisis of the national health service in the former Soviet republics caused a sudden drop in the vaccinations which led to the reappearance of a devastating epidemic of diphtheria, the most important in the last 30 years in developed countries. In the two decades prior to 1990, diphtheria was under control in the Soviet Union, with the rate in the middle of the 1970s similar to that in North

America: in 1975 only 199 cases (0.08 out of 100,000) were recorded and 198 the following year. The infections oscillated around very limited numbers until 1990, when there were 1431 cases: a hike of 70% with respect to the previous year, with a high concentration in the cities of Moscow and Oblast (for a total of 541 cases). In 1991, there were 3126 infections and the epidemic reached St Petersburg, Ukraine and Kiev, reaching 5744 infections in 1992. The real pandemic exploded in 1993, when diphtheria affected 19,462 people (an increase of 290%) in Russia, Ukraine and Belarus. However, it did not spread to Estonia, thanks to an effective vaccination campaign. The following year, there were 50,412 cases, with a maximum rate (two-thirds) of adolescents. Between 1995 and 1996 alone, the cases started to drop, due to a massive intervention of vaccinal prophylaxis. At the end of the epidemic, extensive epidemiological literature confirmed that there had been 150,000 cases of diphtheria and that it had cost the lives of 45,000 people, representing over 90% of all the victims recorded in the world in the period 1990–1995 (Galazka and Dittmann 2000).[19] In this case too, alongside the drop in vaccines other causes are attributed to the deaths—such as cardiovascular diseases, alcoholism and the high murder rate—linked to the difficult political-economic transition of the period (Leon et al. 1997).

Another exemplary case occurred in India between 2009 and 2011, a period of time—when the nation went from having almost half the cases of polio in the world, to zero cases (for 4 years running, until 2015)—which is so short as to exclude from the list of causes any improvements in health and hygiene or socio-economic conditions. It was all thanks to a vaccination campaign that cost more than 41 billion, strongly supported by the Bill and Melinda Gates Foundation. We could also mention the cases, discussed earlier, of the outbreaks of epidemics of whooping cough (1974–1983) and smallpox (2012–2013), due to the decrease in vaccinations in England, which is certainly not a country subject to variations in the hygienic and economic conditions that can justify the spread of epidemics. Going back to Russia, perhaps the most emblematic fact concerns the well-being and longevity that vaccines can offer a population: with the hecatomb of human lives caused by the HIV epidemic which spread in Africa towards the end of the 1980s, the Russian epidemic of diphtheria is the only case in the twentieth century where, in a developed country, there was a clear decrease in life expectancy after decade of continuous growth. This was a traumatic phenomenon which

---

[19] Vitek, C.R. and M. Wharton, Diphtheria in the Former Soviet Union: Reemergence of a Pandemic Disease, "CDC", Vol. 4, No. 4, December 1998, http://tinyurl.com/z65ftdv (the site of the North American CDC lists 63 papers which analyse all the data in detail).

earned ample literature and the technical definition of *Russian epidemiological crisis*. HIV and diphtheria are two infectious diseases and the fact that their spread in a few years was the only health event to have abruptly decreased the longevity and life expectancy in two regions of the world in the twentieth century ought to make the authors of the main Italian websites who deny the importance of vaccines and belittle the risk of infectious diseases reflect seriously.[20]

## Prejudices and Ideologies: Weakening the Immune System

Nature is neither good nor bad; it is simply indifferent to human fate; this is a concept which is obvious for many, but not for everyone. Anyone who has studied biology knows very well that human beings share the planet with a large number of other living organisms, with which they have to share food resources and vital spaces, in a continuous fight for existence. To interpret this relationship, the historian of medicine and doctor Mirko Grmek borrowed the notion of *biocenosis* (which in ecology characterizes all the organisms present in an ecosystem) and suggested the concept of *pathocenosis*, or all the pathological states in a given population at a given time. It is a useful concept to understand the frequency and distribution of infectious diseases, in relation to the dynamics of balance between organisms in the different ecosystems. In a stable ecological situation, the pathocenosis is in a state of balance, with a small number of very frequent diseases and a vast number of rare diseases. If, however, this balance is altered, modifications are created in the relations of force between the organisms which open the way to the spread of infectious agents (Grmek 1985). In the past, the phenomenon of the domestication of plants and animals and the consequent urbanization which started in prehistory to then be consolidated in the Middle Ages, meant going, in a short time, from life in small groups in isolated villages to life in highly populated cities. During this passage, epidemics found an ideal ecological context to spread (we will return to the meaning that these evolutionary aspects have for vaccination and immunity in Chap. 5). In the twentieth century, especially in Western countries, we have seen the eradication of infectious diseases and at the same time the onset of chronic-degenerative ones (such as diabetes, senile dementia and arthrosis) caused by a sudden change in social, economic and

---

[20] The best known are: comilva.org, condav.it, autismovaccini.com, infovaccini.it, mednat.org, vaccinareinformati.org, disinformazione.it, scienzaverde.it.

health conditions which, for the first time in the history of evolution, has made the generalized spread of phenomena such as hypernutrition and a sedentary lifestyle possible. The concept of pathocenosis also suggests the fragility of the present ecological situation. The severe epidemic of haemorrhagic fever caused by the Ebola virus which in 2014 affected Africa and alarmed the whole world was triggered by contacts between the local populations of some regions in central Africa—in all probability the Congo, where the virus was isolated in 1976—and the reservoir organisms that host more or less asymptomatically the virus (like fruit bats or the animals that came into contact with their faeces, such as pigs and monkeys) and infect humans: thanks to air transport, it may only be a short step from African villages to planetary diffusion. The same applies to the fragile balance that exists today in the West between infectious agents and vast and densely populated metropolitan areas.

Germs and men have been confronting one another for thousands of years and after an infinite series of defeats, it was not until the last century that the latter had the better over the former. We must not forget that it is an apparent period of calm: viruses and bacteria have not disappeared; they are only under control, thanks to vaccines and good hygienic conditions. We have seen this in the various "natural experiments" which unfortunately in recent decades have occurred spontaneously in advanced countries (United Kingdom, United States, Russia), where epidemic outbreaks of whooping cough, measles and diphtheria have broken out due to a "simple" decrease in the vaccinal cover. If in Western culture, aided by generalized well-being, that portion of the population who opposes vaccines and pharmacological therapies develops, it will inevitably be destined to succumb with respect, for example, to the emerging Asian cultures, notoriously more disciplined in relation to the institutions—including health regulations. The state of health of a population is similar to that of its rights, which cannot be taken for granted and definitively acquired, but have to be monitored and defended, because they risk being lost every day. In the last quarter of the twentieth century unfortunately, vaccines have been the victim of their success, of that well-being which they allowed by eliminating the major fatal or debilitating infectious diseases which had been the scourge of humanity since their appearance on the earth. This attitude is without any doubt the result of the short memory from one generation to another, a series of social changes and the cognitive biases mentioned in the previous chapters. There is, however, more.

The biological-evolutionary overview of the role of vaccines just mentioned—which is not a personal opinion but a fact supported by a great deal of historical and experimental evidence—inevitably eludes the anti-vaccinationists. They often harbour mixed feelings between exaltation for "natural things" and naturist lifestyles and the cognitive refusal (or even the profound discredit) towards what is produced by humans and industry. Looking closely, it is a naïve and one-sided conception of nature or, better of an ideology focused on an anti-modernist, Luddite and backward idea that looks with nostalgia at bygone times, full of natural food and fresh air, and without chemical agents and toxic drugs. Such an approach, to be clear, must not be confused with the idea—completely rational and that can be agreed with—that respects the environment, natural resources and other animal species. It is, however, one thing to respect nature and another to be subjected to it, embracing the prejudice that everything that it produces is good or better than human things. It is neither good nor bad (but, rather blind), so nature must be chosen case by case, and not without criticism and with prejudices. Let's look at the reasons why.

If we ask which were the most traumatic events of the twentieth century in terms of losses of human lives, most people will think of the victims of the two World Wars. Quite rightly, the collective memory recalls the traumas of the two conflicts as the result of that crazy and self-destructive part of the human mind that put science and technology at the service of weapons of mass destruction, first with poisonous gases (pyprite, phosgene), flamethrowers, armoured tanks, aircraft and submarines and subsequently with the atomic bomb and concentration camps. These events caused 16 million deaths in the first conflict and 70 million in the second. Yet, alongside these facts produced by man, there was a natural event which mowed down perhaps more victims than the two wars put together and which is rarely remembered: the pandemic of "Spanish flu" which in the 2 years from 1918 to 1920 alone caused between 50 and 100 million deaths all over the world (Johnson and Mueller 2002). Recent molecular studies have shown that the influenza virus was the H1N1, a particularly aggressive form of swine influenza which develops in intensive pig farms and can make a dangerous "leap of species" infecting human beings, who have to cope with a pathogen of animal origin unknown to them.

With Spanish flu, nature was able to cut down more victims in 2 years than the world's technical-scientific innovations in 10. Yet, while the multitudes of commentators ready to recall the dangerousness of progress and the consequent need for the principle of precaution are increasingly large and fierce, those who remember to look at nature with rationality and circumspection are few or non-existent. This cognitive attitude is a very common bias, also confirmed by the interesting studies by Dan Kahan in the field of the neurocognitive approach to law. In his research, Kahan finds a preference of society (and also of some scientists) in preferring and remembering the risks produced by man rather than those caused by natural events, in general perceived as more acceptable (Kahan et al. 2009, 2011). Similar cognitive biases make us forget how the risk of a new Spanish flu is not at all improbable, as suggested by data. After the first pandemic, the WHO started to monitor bird and pig farms, because these turned out to be the main reservoirs where the highly pathogenic strains dangerous for man evolve. As in the case of the H5N1 bird flu—which appeared with a number of epidemics in 1957, 1968 and in 2003 in South-East Asia (affecting 150 million birds)—in the case of the H1N1 swine influenza, there was a return in 2009 of a global epidemic which caused 14,000 infections.[21]

To evaluate the distortion of judgement of our perception of nature caused by these biases, it may be worthwhile to recall an elementary fact which has already been mentioned: as long as we lived naturally, our average life expectancy stood at around 35 years. Before the arrival of industry, we had crystalline air, cities on a human scale, food collected in the garden at home and natural remedies for diseases. Yet, in this apparently idyllic context, people generally did not live over the age of 40: hardly an appealing result. In addition, the forms of government were almost everywhere top-down or tyrannical and the rights of the majority of the population virtually ignored—not to mention those of religious minorities, the disabled and the various forms of racial, economic, gender minorities or social status existing. Violence, abuse and murder were very common activities and mainly went unpunished. With the assertion of science and technology, which developed in the first forms of democracy in the West, from 1830 the life expectancy started to increase: in the last two centuries, as we have seen, the average length of our lives has tripled and from 35 in many countries the average life expectancy is over 80 (with Italy in second place amongst the longest-lived). Ignoring this data is not only impossible but it is also dangerous and irresponsible. We do not want to oppose the ideology of modernity to that of nature: those who support modernity do not accept it a priori and are aware of the many limits it imposes. It is precisely critical openness, and above all recourse to data, figures and evidence, that suggests continuing along the path of modernization. Of course, raising doubts and respecting the environment, therefore evaluating empirically (and not prejudicially or fideistically) what it offers. Figures, however, speak clearly. We have already seen how, even today, the rates of suicide and life expectancy in the countryside are worse than those for people living in chaotic cities. The attitude of those who follow a fundamentalist naturist philosophy of life, contrary to industrialization, to then use it in an

---

[21] Archives of Briefing Notes, "Pandemic" (H1N1), 2009, http://tinyurl.com/h3rtp88

opportune way, also seems preconceived: this is the typical case of organic food and homeopathy. Very often those who use homeopathic remedies do so to cure minor problems such as colds or food intolerances, but in the case of severe infections, acute pain or cardiovascular disease have recourse to traditional drugs. The same happens with nutrition: with respect to traditional food, organic food has a longer, more expensive and much less efficient production (and covers a market share of less than 5%). Only mass production can succeed in meeting the nutrition of those nine billion people estimated for 2050 and those who choose organic, instead of criticizing, ought to respect the food industry which, obviously against payment, worries about feeding the less affluent, who are the majority. People are free to eat as they like and to treat themselves with the remedies they deem most opportune, but let us not forget that it is possible to have recourse to organic food and to homeopathy only because there exists a generalized well-being created by the traditional food and pharmaceutical industries, and when there are health or economic difficulties it is possible to use their products. In this sense, some naturist attitudes can be interpreted as the result of a well-being which at times forgets the principle of coherence and of reality.

This is the framework of conceptual reference to which the naturist approach of some anti-vaccinationists belongs. Their aversion to vaccines is part of an attitude of trust in the natural course of biological phenomena, infections included, and in a more generalized criticism of conventional medical and health treatments which use traditional drugs, deemed toxic and ineffective. The social risks of these attitudes (especially if integrated in an institutionalized, educational and social-health model for teaching in schools) will be analysed in the next chapter. Here, it is important to analyse the cultural context which makes possible a distortion of judgement on the functioning of children's immune system.

The conceptual alliance between the anti-vaccine movements and alternative and naturist treatments, in particular homeopathy, has a long tradition that dates back to the nineteenth century. James Compton Burnett (1840–1901), a British doctor who trained in Vienna and Glasgow, and one of the pioneers of modern homeopathy, described the vaccination of smallpox in homeopathic terms in 1884, observing how both therapeutic systems were based on the already mentioned principle of sympathy, whereby "like cures like" and therefore on the idea that the inoculation of a minimum quantity of a pathogenic substance would have induced in the patient a principle of treatment (Burnett 1884). Burnett was a rare case of a homeopath in favour of vaccinations: in a few years, the anti-vaccine movements found in homeopathy an approach contrary to vaccination and more in line with their rejection of the authority of traditional medicine, advocated by the laws of the state (as we have seen in Chap. 2). Things have not changed very much since then. As we will see in the next chapter, various studies on the European population confirm a close relationship between anti-vaccinationism and adhesion to alternative or complementary medicines (Yaqub et al. 2014; Zuzak et al. 2008). This relationship is particularly solid amongst the radical opponents of vaccinations (Hobson-West 2007). In Canada, one of the sources that persuades parents to develop ideas against vaccinations is the information delivered by those who practise alternative medicine (Busse et al. 2005; Greenberg et al. 2017), which is also confirmed by a recent analysis conducted in Australia (Chow et al. 2017). Similarly, in the United States, parents who have recourse to naturopaths during the vaccinal age of their children (ages 1–7) have offspring with a low rate of vaccination (Downey et al. 2010). In Italy as well, the most extreme group against vaccinations, defined *group of critical parents* (equal to 8.4% of parents), is that "much more inclined, compared with other groups, to use non-conventional medicine as a strategy of prevention" with a percentage of 27.4 and with 35.7% who say that they have used it in the last 12 months.[22]

Specifically, the mistrust that a large part of naturists and homeopaths have for vaccinations rests on the mistaken belief that they weaken the immune system. The basic mechanisms of the immune system, however, reveal a different reality, based on some principles that are not so far from those proposed by naturists and homeopaths. Let's have a look at the two main ones. The immune system is characterized by the ability to "recognize" the molecules outside its body and, therefore, potentially harmful and to keep a cellular "memory" of these encounters. This is how immunization takes place: an infectious agent that is deactivated, dead or crushed in its significant parts (immunogenic), is inoculated and once in circulation it is recognized as external and attacked by the cells which, after a series of reactions, produce antibodies that can neutralize the invader. When it is eliminated, the cells which have produced the efficient antibodies continue to reproduce in time, even for decades: if the infectious agent were to return they are already to attack it, thus avoiding the infection appearing again. This is the artificial immunity acquired by vaccination. To have lifetime cover, some vaccines require one or more inoculations close together, such as the one against yellow fever, hepatitis A and B or polio (OPV). On the other hand, others need a booster dose after some years (e.g. against tetanus and diphtheria), but the principles of *recognition and memory* at the basis of the concept of immunity

---

[22] Censis. Cultura della vaccinazione in Italia: un'indagine sui genitori, October 2014, p. 101.

are the same. There is another fundamental concept to understand immunity and it is *specificity*: it consists of the fact that every time we subject the same infectious agent to immune cells, their response is increasingly adapted and specific to the surface of the invader. This is because in time the antibodies adapt and fit increasingly well with the antigens of the infectious agent. If we observe the diagrams of antibody production, between the first, the second and the third inoculation of a pathogenic agent into the blood, we can see that the quantity and the quality of the antibodies increase incredibly: they are like an army which is specialized and reinforced every time it meets the enemy. From this point of view, it should emerge clearly how the immune system has evolved, precisely to be stimulated to remember, and the memory, although it is understood differently, is a central notion of homeopathy as well. It is, therefore, nonsense to believe that vaccines weaken the immune system; if anything, they reinforce it. This means that if we take two children, one vaccinated several times and one never, and the difference of their "soldier-antibodies" is measured, we discover inevitably that the army of the first child is much larger, diversified from the point of view of the enemies they can deal with and specialized in fighting techniques. If we base ourselves on data and incontrovertible experimental evidence, there can be no doubts at all about the fact that children who have not been vaccinated are at greater risk of contracting infectious diseases and, consequently, they will be weaker than children who have been vaccinated.

This explanation, which takes on greater value if we adopt an evolutionary point of view, is based on the well-known *hygiene hypothesis*. According to this hypothesis, children who, during the phases of their development, have not been sufficiently exposed to infectious agents, intestinal microorganisms of the bacterial flora and parasites tend to develop allergic and autoimmune diseases more frequently at a mature age. The central idea is that in conditions of great hygiene, the immune system in the first years of life does not correctly develop immunological tolerance (the fourth and last concept to understand the basics of immune reactions) or the capacity to remember and ignore the cellular surfaces and the molecules with which it came into contact at an early age. This is a fundamental phenomenon for the purposes of our survival: if the immune system of each individual did not develop a tolerance towards its own body, it would be recognized as "external" and attacked and destroyed by the anti-bodies—just as happens in self-immune diseases, where the individual becomes immunologically auto-intolerant. In other words, if, when we are small, our immune system is not sufficiently stimulated to be diversified towards various external aggressors, it will tend to direct its production of antibodies towards the internal tissues. This pathology can lead to asthmatic pathologies and allergic rhinitis, if contracted in mild forms, but even type 1 diabetes and severe autoimmune diseases in the most serious cases. The hypothesis was put forward by David P. Strachan in 1989, after having observed how the twentieth century had been characterized by a low rate of infantile infections and an increase in allergic diseases. Subsequent studies showed that the youngest siblings in large families, unlike the firstborn children, rarely showed asthmatic allergies; a promiscuous hygienic environment and the infectious diseases of the elder siblings stimulated the immune system of the youngest ones, avoiding future allergic problems for them. There soon emerged a correlation between the excessive attention to hygiene, the prerogative of the higher socio-economic classes and the greater rate of allergic pathologies shown by their offspring. The key concept of these theories is that the immune system is not stable in time, but evolves according to the biography of each individual, or according to the environments lived in, the stimulations perceived and the diseases contracted; it reshapes in time its adaptive responses (Grignolio 2010; Grignolio et al. 2014). A further evolutionary explanation of the hygiene theory, called *old friends hypothesis*, believes that in the Neolithic age our immune system began to coevolve with the parasites to which we were exposed on a daily basis (helminths, small worms and viruses), and that this cohabitation created significant adaptations, including the immune system's need to constantly fight aggression by infectious agents. This training to produce antibodies has lasted for thousands of years, and it has only been for a few decades that, so to speak, it has been forced to go round in circles due to the absence, or near absence, of germs: an evolutionary anomaly that can lead to allergic or autoimmune diseases.

This brief biological-evolutionary overview helps us clearly understand how the fears of naturists that the immune system is weakened are nonsense.

# 4

# How to Unmask the Anti-vaccination "Experts"

## Alternative Philosophies: Homeopaths, Naturists and Steiner

"Talk to the mothers of ill children, look at the suffering in their faces, there are very many cases that science ignores". When you hear words like that, you had better start to worry; they are typical of those who, having recourse to the instrumental use of the emotions and supposed limits of the scientific method, advocate alternative therapeutic treatments to traditional medicine. Concern ought to start from the observation that these treatments are ineffective because something like "alternative medicine", as opposed to "traditional medicine", does not exist. Rather, medicine exists, with its data, its evidence, standard protocols and its rules of validation for drugs and therapies which even includes the use of experimental protocols for innovative therapies, the efficacy of which, partially shown, requires further proof. Outside this form of medicine there is no other medicine, simply there is nothing. This is why the expression "alternative treatments" is used, to clarify the fact that they have nothing to do with confirmed or experimental clinical therapies. The advocates of alternative treatments, in general, refuse these arguments, accusing doctors and scientists of being without a "mental openness" but this is another false argument: mental openness consists not of accepting opinions only because they are alternative to consolidated theories but remaining open to all the hypotheses or criticisms possible, on condition that they are based on data that can be proven. Mental openness is measured on facts, never on personal

© Springer International Publishing AG, part of Springer Nature 2018
A. Grignolio, *Vaccines: Are they Worth a Shot?*, https://doi.org/10.1007/978-3-319-68106-1_4

opinions—otherwise the risk is that of returning to magic or to witchcraft. Let's look at the reasons why.

The opponents of vaccinations always use the argument of personal experience. Let's take the case of a paediatrician who has doubts about the efficacy of vaccinations (a tiny minority, we have seen, much less than 1%): their rhetorical strategy consists of relating their own experiences, built up on stories of patients who have had adverse reactions to the vaccine or particularly healthy patients who have never been vaccinated. In general, alongside these cases, the accounts of the families of patients are related, according to the well-known strategy of *person-centred narrative technique* (Betsch et al. 2012), which naturally corroborate the theories against vaccinations. These are, however, inadmissible criticisms—especially if maintained by a doctor who ought to know the foundations of the experimental method—because they ignore that modern medicine comes into being precisely to oppose this type of individual experience. In other words, a doctor who were to realize the harmfulness or inefficacy of vaccines during his examinations should be the first to doubt such phenomena which go completely against the knowledge acquired, based on hundreds of thousands of pieces of data collected by colleagues. If, out of pure scruple—as moreover takes place occasionally in literature—he wanted to measure the effective harmfulness or inefficacy of vaccines, the way is not to sign petitions to the public authorities or advertise himself becoming credited as a doctor who doubts vaccinations, but rather to start a controlled clinical trial. Every human being has accumulated a series of experiences during their professional life: some have general validity, others represent simple isolated cases without significance and subjective perception or personal conviction is certainly not the right instrument to distinguish between them. This is why before inventing the scientific method there were esoteric attitudes typical of magic, that is, as many theories and treatments as there were practising doctors: each one with their therapy, valid according to their followers and the ability of treatment of these theories on average did not allow passing the threshold of the age of 40. Science came into being precisely to emerge from this chaos of subjective convictions, thanks to six marvellous instruments which have allowed making some knowledge objectively valid and eliminating others as false or irrelevant. It was only with these instruments that the rigorous medical science that we know today developed in the twentieth century and has allowed saving millions of lives.

The first instrument is the *experimental clinical study*, also known as *clinical trial*, which consists of recruiting a certain number of subjects on whom to test a new therapy, for example for the administration of a drug, in order to collect data and evaluate both its safety (and therefore exclude any harmfulness) and its efficacy. The second instrument requires this trial to be *controlled*, a technical term that refers to the need to divide the sample of subjects of a clinical trial into two groups: one that receives the treatment and one (called the *control group*) that receives a different one (or none) so that, if the experimentation is carried out correctly, the two groups are homogeneous and the effects comparable. The third rule is that the assignment of the individuals to one of the two groups is *randomized*, i.e. casual, so that any other variables which are not the object of study are distributed uniformly and the differences between the two groups are to be attributed to the treatment (in actual fact, randomization is only one of the various statistical instruments to make the sample reliable). The fourth, and perhaps the best known, instrument is the introduction of the *placebo*, a fake pharmacological treatment (a tablet of sugar) which is indistinguishable from a real one: it is used to eliminate the distortions due to the expectations present both in the patients who wish to recover, accentuating the positive symptoms, and in the researchers who tend to consider the data confirming their hypotheses and to neglect contrasting data. The fifth instrument is the *double blind*, which prohibits both the experimenters and the patients from knowing which is the placebo and which is the drug. Lastly, the sixth instrument concerns the different procedures of *peer review*, which go from the first control by the editors of the scientific journal in which the study will be published, to the revision of the data and the control of the methodological appropriateness, the solidity of the results presented and the reliability of the conclusions. All these activities are carried out by a series of colleagues who are experts in the disciplinary sector and known as *peers*: anonymous third parties who are independent and competent and can ask (as often occurs) for further experiments and verifications. In addition, when the findings have been published, there are the criticisms or mentions of support that scientific literature produces to corroborate the study or not.

As can clearly be seen, science is perfectly aware of the human tendency to distortions of subjective judgement, from which scientists are by no means exempt and the counter-measures necessary to eliminate them from the experimental clinical trials (as clearly chosen in the case of the placebo effect and double blind). Scientists know these involuntary mechanisms only too well and are the first to want to protect their research from any procedural flaws in order to obtain solid research, based on verifiable data and evidence, as well as reproducible by anyone else: this is how scientific knowledge has been produced for at least a century and this is how scientific knowledge advances all over the world. The intentional refusal to submit to experimental investigation one's personal clinical-therapeutic opinions is a different matter and this is effectively what happens in that minority of doctors who side with the anti-vaccinationists.

We have seen how in the United States the percentage of doctors who are against vaccination is numerically insignificant (0.02%). It is not a coincidence that, as in other European countries, they also generally have specializations which have little to do with vaccines and immunology. Browsing through their profiles, they are mainly homeopaths, psychiatrists, surgeons and often add to their specialization adjectives which inform us of their "alternative" approach to traditional medicine, such as "holistic", "supplementary" or "functional", all of which are approaches which tend not to be based on scientific evidence. The same applies to anti-vaccinationist parents, to whom they offer "technical" consulting services; in the United States as well, these doctors vary their criticisms, going from radical anti-vaccination positions, like those who express themselves in favour of the vaccine and autism relationship, to those apparently more nuanced ones, who deem that infectious diseases contracted naturally are an excellent natural remedy to acquire immunity. In both cases, measles is often at the centre of the attention of the criticisms. It is in this context that "measles-parties" have caught on in the united States and in Europe organized, often with the help of social networks, by anti-vaccination and naturist parents to allow the spread of the natural form of the measles virus, erroneously deemed more acceptable because it is "natural". In California, this irresponsible practice has spread so much in recent years that it has driven some anti-vaccinationist parents to send by post lollipops or clothes used by children with measles. This is a very dangerous procedure—due to the high pathogenicity (on average one person every 2000–3000 who are infected dies) and contagiousness of the virus (one infected person infects on average 16–18 other people)—has made the American authorities stress that it is illegal to use public or private postal services to send infected material (Ghianni 2011; Brown 2011). The same practice also became popular in Germany and in 2015, an 18-month-old child died, in a dramatic episode which in this case too involved the political and health authorities, making them evaluate different forms of raising social awareness about the importance of vaccinations (Knight 2015).

In Italy as well, the letter-petition of 2015, already mentioned, by anti-vaccinationist doctors—two of whom in 2017 were struck off the medical register, while one has been temporarily suspended from exercising the profession, following their repeated public calls against vaccinations—is focused on the anti-measles vaccine and on the beneficial effects of natural infections. The text is based on the idea that paediatric vaccinations are harmful due to their adverse reactions and capacity to weaken the children's immune system, through the hyperstimulation caused by multiple vaccines and by the toxicity of adjuvants and preservatives. Alongside this main idea, other concepts are expressed, typical of anti-vaccinationist thought and already present in nineteenth century criticisms: for example, children who are not vaccinated "appear undoubtedly and globally healthier", that "today children are immunologically weaker than children of the same age a few decades ago" and that the medicine of the future "can certainly not be based on the use of drugs, but first of all on a correct hygiene of life". No scientific research is quoted to support these "theories" but only the personal experiences of the two doctors who drew up the letter and these experiences are reported with expressions such as "it is well known that", "we have realized that", "it is a fact that comes from daily clinical experience", "evidence that any attentive and observant doctor can notice", "these 35–40 years of specialized medical practice alongside the ill child, not hasty but consisting of observing and listening, of considering what he communicates to us and subliminally [sic] and what the parents tell us, has opened our eyes . . ." These arguments, as can be seen, are inconsistent from an experimental point of view. The letter addressed to the President of the Istituto Superiore di Sanità ends with a series of suggestions, including: superseding the vaccinal obligation by law, freedom by parents and the paediatrician not to vaccinate their children, the request for individual vaccines and postponing the age of administration. Lastly, the authors appeal (taking care not to quote them) to the "fierce debates in scientific circles" expressed by the scientific community and relaunched by parents concerning vaccinations and they conclude referring to the 120 signatures of the subscribers of the appeal and the "very many Doctors and Associations that agree with these concepts." Browsing through the signatures, as in the lists of US anti-vaccinationist doctors, a massive presence of medical specialities which do not have a great deal to do with vaccinations can be noticed (urologists, psychiatrists, psychotherapists, cardiologists, nutritionists, etc.); there is no vaccinologist or epidemiologist or immunologist. There are, however, 22 paediatricians, the profession which returns with the greatest frequency in the text, conveying the (false) idea that they are, for the most part, contrary to vaccinations: the paediatric associations have not only always been the most active in vigorously supporting their extreme importance but a number of studies show that it is paediatricians themselves, of all the categories of doctors, who administer the greatest number of vaccinations to their children (Posfay-Barbe et al. 2005; Martin and Badalyan 2012).

In essence, it is a letter which can be taken as a model of the typical anti-scientist attitude. The rhetorical strategy is always the same: to raise general doubts spread by the Internet avoiding bringing data and evidence, reporting personal clinical experiences and those of the parents of ill children, to appeal to the press and the political institutions instead of the competent bodies and scientific journals and lastly, throw discredit on the authority of traditional medicine—perceived as narrow and oppressive—to which a naturist lifestyle and greater empathy with nature are opposed. The inconsistency of all these topics has already been dealt with in the previous chapter.

However, one point of the letter can be analysed, as it is not only the central theory of the appeal but it is a critical position shared, as mentioned, by other US and European anti-vaccinationist doctors. It is the idea that children who are not vaccinated are "undoubtedly and globally healthier, less subject to infectious pathologies", unlike children who are given the trivalent MMR vaccination, which the authors believe is "in scientific literature, especially in the USA" currently at the centre of "heated discussion on the risk/benefit ratio". They are, therefore, "willing to take part in a study [. . .] which compared in the strictest way possible the state of health of children completely vaccinated with that of children who have not been vaccinated". As chance would have it, this study was carried out and published in 2014 in the American journal "Science", one of the most authoritative in the world. The authors of this important study show that the vaccination against measles has several benefits, which go well beyond those known to date. Analysing a huge amount of data from the national epidemiological data of England, Wales, the United States and Denmark, which cover the years from 1950—when measles were common and the trivalent MMR had not yet been introduced—to 2010, the authors have shown how the vaccination for measles is associated with the decrease of infant mortality, confirming some previous studies on smaller samples (Goldhaber-Fiebert et al. 2010; McBride 2015). The action on the immune system of the naturally contracted virus, the study explains, causes severe immunosuppression in infected people (due to the decrease of lymphocytes B and T) capable of altering the immunological memory for 2–3 years, the period which exposes the subjects to opportunistic fatal infections not linked to measles. The population data of the historical series confirm, both in the previous era and in the one following the introduction of the vaccine for measles, a high rate of infant mortality from infectious diseases in the delicate period of post-measles convalescence. For this reason, the study concludes the observation of the data of the last 60 years and shows that the vaccination against measles is a fundamental preventive treatment, which not only does not weaken children but makes them healthier and gives them a greater life expectancy compared to children who are not vaccinated (Mina et al. 2014).

This letter-appeal signed by 120 Italian doctors is not the only anti-vaccination drive inside medical knowledge: as shown also by the Censis

2014 report, in the various disciplines and amongst the ranks of healthcare operators, there is a doubtful minority regarding paediatric vaccinations. This observation shows that in Italy, among the various voices that "explicitly do not advise the recommended (not compulsory) vaccinations in paediatric age" to parents, after 28.4% represented by "friends and acquaintances", there are 18% represented by doctors (GPs and specialists) and healthcare operators (obstetricians, nurses and other personnel).[1] Several international studies suggest that the majority of the small, but influential, portion of healthcare operators is mainly made up of obstetricians and nurses, to the point that in Australia, for example, the competent authorities decided to issue an official statement in 2016 in which severe measures of penalties and controls are issued for operators who dissuade (including through the social media) patients from being vaccinated, reminding its members of their adhesion to standard practices based on evidence of efficacy (Zhang et al. 2011; Gallant et al. 2009; Wicker and Rose 2011; Ryser and Heininger 2015; Dube et al. 2013).[2] It has to be specified that, although indirectly and involuntarily, it is the low adhesion by healthcare operators to programmes of vaccinal prophylaxis that also fuels fears on vaccinations. This is an irresponsible attitude which for years has made the European authorities ask whether it is opportune or not to make them compulsory for such a category at risk, considering their contact with patients who are potentially contagious or immunosuppressed (La Torre et al. 2009; Galanakis et al. 2013, 2014). The most alarming data, as mentioned, emerges from a number of studies which, in recent years, have revealed the dangerous presence of some areas of resistance from homeopathic doctors and supporters of the anthroposophic approach common in Steiner schools. Let's have a look at these.

From the mid-1990s, when the first studies aimed at observing the reasons underlying the rejection of vaccines started, an English study published in the "British Medical Journal" revealed that over 50% of parents who did not have their children vaccinated did so by appealing to homeopathic medicine. Even then, the fears of parents reported by the survey accused multiple vaccinations of being capable of "causing autoimmune diseases or weakening the immune system" and they aimed at "reinforcing the defences of the organism through excellent nutrition, good hygiene and letting the body contract the normal

---

[1] Censis, Cultura della vaccinazione in Italia: un'indagine sui genitori, October 2014, Tab. 17 and 18, pp. 81–82.

[2] Nursing and Midwifery Board of Australia. Position statement on nurses, midwives and vaccination—October 2016: https://goo.gl/kVYzcJ

form of the disease without suppressing it", not believing therefore "the risk of the disease greater than that of the vaccination" (Simpson et al. 1995). Subsequent studies delved deeper into these data, reporting how only 23% of Austrian homeopaths deemed immunization important and it was discovered that other "alternative medicines" and naturopathic approaches similarly discredited vaccinations (Ernst 1995). The epidemiological studies which followed the Wakefield affair to monitor the decrease in the trivalent MMR vaccine also found in the parents of children who had not been vaccinated or partially vaccinated, a clear adhesion to homeopathic practices (Schmidt and Ernst 2002), with data of particular concern in Switzerland, Germany and Canada (Zuzak et al. 2008; Gnadinger et al. 2009; Schonberger et al. 2009; Rieder and Robinson 2015). According to some authors, the spread of homeopathy is putting the decline in vaccinal cover at even greater risk, to the extent that the anti-vaccination movements often refer—about 90% of websites—to this practice as a base for its methodological assumptions and to build up arguments against vaccinations (Ernst 2001; Davidovitch 2004; Blume 2006; Kata 2010). This relationship is today so consolidated that it is not even scathed by the appeals and by the declarations of principle which (rarely) the associations of homeopathic doctors issue to their members in support of vaccinations. Even when it is not the homeopaths who do not recommend vaccinations, this therapeutic approach is, in any case, the one preferred by the parents of children who have not been vaccinated (Kriwy 2011). It is, therefore, a vicious circle that is potentially dangerous for public health.

The anthroposophic medicine common in Steiner schools deserves a separate discussion. Anthroposophy is an alternative and esoteric medicine which originated around the figure of the Austrian philosopher and educationalist Rudolf Steiner (1861–1925). It spread in the twentieth century initially in Switzerland and Germany and then in the rest of Europe. Recovering some themes of German romanticism, the anthroposophy of Steiner focuses on a spiritual dimension based on mystical inspiration, the imagination and intuition. It also aimed at merging the world of visible things and the natural and supernatural forces and energies, a correspondence best expressed by *eurythmy*—an art which aspires, through gestures and movements, to make visible what lives in secret in words and in music. Steiner applied these concepts to different areas of knowledge such as education (Steiner or Waldorf), medicine (anthroposophic) and agriculture (biodynamic). In the last named, practised and taught in the schools, for example, to keep the matter-vital force useful for fertilizing, it is fundamental to alternate sprays of ground quartz with the rite of *horn manure*, the horn of a cow (which has calved at least once) filled with dung at a certain phase of the full moon. Anthroposophic medicine, although it declares it is not opposed to conventional medicine, shares a number of aspects with naturopathy and homeopathy—including rejecting vaccinations and mistrust of antibiotics and antipyretics—and is particularly sensitive to natural food and to the spiritual dimension of diseases. Steiner or Waldorf education developed from the school founded by Steiner in 1919 to offer an education to the children of the clerks at the Waldorf-Astoria tobacco factory in Stuttgart: the primary aim of this education, at least in the intentions, consists of encouraging the pupils to develop, with different mystical touches, independent, creative, socially responsible and compassionate thought. There are estimated to be more than one thousand Steiner schools in the world today (which cover education from the nursery to secondary school), seven hundred of which are in Europe, with about thirty in Italy.

The combination of these educational principles and similar habits (in part already present in some parents before school enrolment) makes the Steiner schools a free port for vaccinal prophylaxis, where in all probability there are the lowest levels of herd immunity in Western culture—and where numerous and severe outbreaks of epidemics have been recorded in the past 15 years, amply discussed by scientific literature. In Europe, the first significant case emerged in the United Kingdom, where in 2000 a series of infections of measles were recorded. They could be traced to an "anthroposophic community in London". The authorities concentrated their attention on a first group of thirty children, and in the following months the number of pupils affected rose to 293, 90% of whom were under 15. 87% of them had not been vaccinated against measles, because it was deemed an "ineffective and unsafe" practice and in any case capable of blocking the "reinforcing beneficial effect" for the development in the children of the natural course of the disease (Hanratty et al. 2000; Duffell 2001). Between 1999 and 2000 in the Netherlands, there was an even more dramatic epidemic: 3292 cases of children affected by measles, of whom 94% had not been vaccinated; the parents of 100 of them opposed vaccinations, stating "anthroposophic beliefs". Out of the total, 16% had severe complications and there were three deaths (Van den Hof et al. 2006). In 2008, there was another outbreak of a measles epidemic in the Netherlands, again in the anthroposophic community: at first there were 34 cases in the Hague and another 2 infections in Leiderdorp and Utrecht. The authorities discovered that the first patient (the *index case*) was an "8-year-old child enrolled in a school of 210 pupils" many of whom came from an anthroposophic community where the parents were opposed to vaccines". In a few days, nine other cases were recorded in the school, while later, there was a second infectious strain in the anthroposophic community of the Hague from which it emerged that, out of the 34 infected children, 31 had not been vaccinated (Van Velzen et al. 2008). The first known Austrian case dates back to 2008, when 392 cases of measles were recorded, of which 168 came from the anthroposophic community. Subsequent analyses in the school where the epidemic had developed revealed perhaps something unique in the European school panorama: only 0.6% of the pupils enrolled had been vaccinated (Schmid et al. 2010). Lastly, the three German epidemics must be mentioned. The first was in 2003, when in a Steiner school in Coburg, in upper Bavaria, there were 1191 cases of measles among the pupils, of whom only 9% had been vaccinated: 28% of those infected had "severe complications" (Arenz et al. 2003; Ernst 2011). Between March and May 2010 there was a second epidemic in the Essen district, in Rhine-Westphalia, which appeared with 71 cases of measles and 4 hospitalizations, "the majority coming from a Waldorf school". The German authorities intervened promptly, preventing the non-immune children from attending school for 2 weeks and establishing that, out of the 71 infected, 30 were from the Steiner kindergarten and school, 18 were their relatives and 20 had gone to doctors belonging to that community and who advised against vaccination. Extensive subsequent controls by the health services showed that, out of the 762 pupils of the Steiner school, 311 (41%) were not vaccinated (Roggendorf et al. 2010). In the same period, Berlin was affected by another infectious strain of measles contracted, during a recent trip to India, by a Steiner student without vaccinal coverage: on his return, the student was able to infect 52 individuals belonging to his school, where less than 70% of the pupils had been vaccinated against measles. Subsequent analyses showed how the spread of the epidemic had selectively attacked pupils with an average age of 10, comprised between 1 and 18, belonging to two Steiner schools in two different parts of the city and then spread to their relatives, but without infecting the non-Steiner schools present in the same areas (Batzing-Feigenbaum et al. 2010). To date, there are no data available on the vaccinal cover of Italian Steiner schools, but there is no reason to think that their situation is significantly different from the European context just mentioned.

A recent and insightful analysis of the situation in the United States shows a context which for certain aspects is similar, but with some significant differences (Sobo 2015). The Steiner schools in North America also show the highest rate of refusal of vaccinations with an average among the pupils of 51%, ten times greater than the 6.1% in private schools and 2.7% in state schools. Even though the anti-vaccination attitude is present in a small part of the parents before enrolment, the majority of the refusals come in the first years of education, for reasons that each time focus on the inefficiency, on the toxicity and on the economic interests alleged to be behind the vaccines. Unlike the European case, however, American parents seem to base their rejection not on anthroposophy but on a strong spirit of adhesion to the shared social rules, according to the model of cultural cognition proposed by Dan Kahan: the parents conform their perception to the predominant one in the group and the community to which they feel they belong (Kahan 2012, 2014)—a similar explanation could have acted on a Somali community in Minnesota which, influenced by an anti-vaccination campaign focused on the autism-trivalent relationship, stopped vaccinating their members causing, between April and May 2017, a worrying infectious outbreak of measles which alerted the scientific community.[3] As in the Italian cases mentioned in the first chapter, many parents of children at Steiner schools in America have a fairly high cultural level and pay particular attention to health topics; therefore, they answer the criticisms on the absence of vaccination by opposing a strong refusal and a greater cognitive closure (Nyhan et al. 2014). Instead of stimulating similar defensive attitudes, the author concludes that a strategy of involving the parents focused on questions shared by the Steiner educational values, such as the common good of society (herd immunity) and the independence and freedom of thought, also applicable to the hygiene-health choices—as well as the presentation of statistics which compare the perception of the risk of vaccination with the risks of play-recreational activities that the children at Steiner schools perform every day in contact with nature—seems to be efficient.

## The "Alternative Therapies": The Charlatan's Script in 5 Points

Alongside the cases discussed in the previous paragraph, there are various cases of shady characters who oppose vaccinations out of pure personal interest. They may be doctors, healthcare operators or experts in "alternative" or "complementary treatments" and have in common the fact of accusing vaccines of the most widely varying pathologies in order to sell their diets, therapies and expensive advice. In the history of medicine and at juridical level, a technical term is used to describe this figure: the *charlatan*. The figure

---

[3] Centers for Disease Control and Prevention (CDC). Morbidity and Mortality Weekly Report (MMWR). Measles Outbreak—Minnesota April–May 2017 Weekly/July 14, 2017/66(27);713–717, Victoria Hall et al. (https://www.cdc.gov/mmwr/volumes/66/wr/mm6627a1.htm).

of the swindler and of the travelling healer capable of seducing market squares has existed stably as a social phenomenon at least since the Renaissance (Gentilcore 2006; Conforti et al. 2012, p. 159) and has come down more or less intact to us today. Few recall, for example, that the most important and authoritative regulatory agency for the control of food and drugs, the U.S. FDA, was set up in 1906 precisely to stem the spread of snake oil, a phony and dangerous treatment offered by charlatans as a panacea for a whole set of diseases which were then common.[4] The main characteristic of the charlatan, even today, consists of offering cures or therapeutic treatments that ordinary medicine cannot or does not yet know how to provide, aware of finding minds weakened by pain, the illusions and hopes of patients and their families. The case of autism is exemplary: having someone who accuses paediatric vaccines of causing autism means for some parents at last finding an external cause on which to blame a disease which is still without a precise aetiological framework. Each fragility of the health service and each failed cure represents a possible terrain of conquest for the charlatan.

Italy, as already mentioned in Chap. 1, has its tradition of charlatans. One case that stands for all is the recent national one of the so-called *Stamina method*, where a presumed "therapy based on stem cells" was sold, at a cost of between 30,000 and 50,000 €, to treat a wide variety of neurodegenerative diseases in adults and children. The tests on the "System cell products" carried out by the NAS [Anti-Sophistication and Health Division] of the Carabinieri revealed the presence of polluted material and doses of stem cells which, when present, were more suitable for rodents than for human beings. If those responsible for this swindle had not exaggerated in their aims by trying to obtain a funding of three million euro from Parliament by way of reimbursement from the National Health Service, and administering the treatment in a well-known public hospital, they might still be active on the market, intent on their fraud to the detriment of popular credulity. The case of the European and North American anti-vaccinationists is not very different, but is in fact more articulated (Chap. 1). There are various charlatans who offer pre- and post-vaccination "detoxing" products and supplements, gluten-free and casein-free diets capable of "healing" autism caused by a vaccine, protocols capable of "curing" intoxications, pathologies of the metabolism or of the gastrointestinal tract responsible for a broad spectrum of mental retardation disorders and, lastly, homotoxicological or "chelating" treatments that are alleged to be

---

[4] U.S. Food and Drug Administration, History, http://tinyurl.com/guhjnnd

able to "detoxify" or restore the activity of the immune system after the "post-vaccination immunosuppression".

As already mentioned several times in this book, history can be of help with its ability to line up events of the past to be able to find any regularities: while different charlatans in Italy and abroad seem to follow a serial fraudulent behaviour. The difference is that abroad, the institutions close the ranks around scientists and competences more tightly and the organs of information, beyond an initial interest for attractive topics on the level of the media, wisely switch off the spotlights on what turn out to be personal dramas capable of igniting dangerous populist fires. Political representatives, the magistrature and television programmes, even only with general competences in the scientific and biomedical field in their staff, would not fall into the sham woven by the charlatan of the moment, and some decisions on the relationship between autism and vaccines, which after having been irresponsibly accepted in the first degrees of judgement were fortunately overturned in the final judgement by the Italian Court of Cassation, could have been avoided.

Here is, in five points, the classic script followed by charlatans to entrap their victims. These points have been constructed starting from recent cases in the news of frauds in the biomedical field. The warning that the great Greek historian, Thucydides, who survived the plague of Athens in 430 BC, gave his readers in the hope of offering instruments to stem future epidemics applies to them: "on my part, I will say how [the disease] appeared and with which symptoms: so that if one day it were to come back and rage again, everyone can be attentive, knowing its characteristics first, and know what it is".

*Rule No. 1. The charlatan of the day is the author of a so-called revolutionary discovery capable of healing diseases which today are incurable, but he is opposed and marginalized by the scientific community.*

This is a nineteenth century literary cliché, also called the *Galileo effect*, which imagines the scientist as an eccentric genius in his laboratory isolated from the world who "sees beyond" his time and is unpopular with the conservative and standardizing scientific community. In the history of science, the figure of the Renaissance scientist Galileo Galilei (1564–1642) is an emblematic figure of the misunderstood genius, capable of subverting scientific knowledge of the time ahead of his times. Applying this cliché to the context of the present day, however, is a vulgar historical error: the story of Galileo dates back 400 years, when there was no scientific community and science was at its beginnings, while today a scientist who puts forward a new theory has all the strategies—validated evidence, experiments and conferences—to convince his colleagues. Research is a collective and international undertaking, anyone can publish data and theories, and the whole community evaluates the worth and reliability of the proposal through the publications of the scientific journals. A new theory or therapy, capable of explaining and healing incurable diseases, is received with enthusiasm and awarded prizes, at times the Nobel prize. Today, it would be more appropriate to speak of the *Einstein factor*, which proves how an unknown boy, working in a marginal patents institute, publishing overwhelming evidence in a scientific journal, can write an article that revolutionizes the laws of physics: what happened to Einstein a century ago reminds us that the only thing that counts in science today is solid evidence, made public and certified by the community of peers. Take the case of the *Helicobacter pylori*, the bacterium that today we know is responsible for peptic ulcers. For decades, it was deemed that the stomach was sterile and that the cause of the ulcer was to be found in the gastric juices, capable of corroding the intestinal mucus if released in excess. All the pharmacological treatments were focused on reducing the acid secretions of the stomach, according to the saying, "no acid, no ulcer". From 1980 onwards, two Australian researchers, Barry J. Marshall and J. Robin Warren, realized that the ulcer could be an infectious disease and started a series of experiments and publications to prove their theory. It was not easy to convince the whole scientific community, but data, evidence and experiments were stronger than any resistance and in 2005 they were awarded the Nobel Prize for medicine and physiology (Van Der Weyden et al. 2005). Twentieth century science is studded with stories like this one.

*Rule No. 2. According to the charlatan, his innovative therapy is opposed by the "powers that be", in particular the pharmaceutical multinational corporations, which have the purpose of not curing patients in order to make greater economic gains from the disease or, depending on the versions, to exclude anyone who is not under their financial control.*

We have already said that the multinationals, like all companies that invest money for a purpose, need an economic return. Virtuous behaviour (e.g. they produce, at often contained costs, lifesaving oncological drugs, or invaluable antibiotics, or donate drugs or funds for research to developing countries) is alternated with less virtuous behaviour (this is the case of the failure to produce "orphan" drugs for rare diseases because they are incapable of producing revenue or the attempts to create cartel agreements to avoid reducing the prices of drugs). Without considering them saints or demons, we can say that they are free enterprises which focus on innovation and profit, just like any small businessman, professional person or any representative of a free enterprise; in this sense—contrary to what the charlatans maintain—the pharmaceutical companies, instead of hindering new therapies, if anything, encourage them. Those who develop an innovative therapy which is certified and patented according to agreed rules also has every interest in receiving funding and aid from the pharmaceutical multinational corporations and from other bodies so that their therapeutic protocol is circulated. Let's take the case of Holoclar (an all-Italian merit) the first drug in the world based on stem cells capable of reconstructing the cornea damaged by burns or trauma. The research was started by only two researchers, Michele De Luca and Graziella Pellegrini, at the University of Modena and Reggio Emilia (research started with public funds) who took more than 10 years to develop their research in one of the most competitive and innovative fields in the world, that of stem cells, and where the financial appetites are, therefore, the greatest. When their research concluded the preclinical experimental phase and they needed funding to go from the laboratory to the patient's bed, the so-called phase of *therapeutic translation*, the researchers decided to work in partnership with a medium-sized pharmaceutical company, the Chiesi group, which built expensive laboratories according to the *Good Manufacturing Practices*, GMP, developed the drug based on stem cells and started the complex regulatory part. The European Medicines Agency (EMA) has recently defined Holoclar one of the milestones in its history and in February 2015 the European Commission issued an authorization for it to be marketed, valid throughout the EU. Holoclar is only one example of the many collaborations between public and private sectors and between individual researchers and pharmaceutical companies, which proves the falsity of the charlatans' arguments.

In general, the accusations they level against the economic interests and the desire to control the market of therapies can, if anything, be addressed to them: it is the charlatan who always and exclusively has commercial interests and the only way to defend a false therapy not based on evidence of its efficacy is to attack authentic competitors in an instrumental and one-sided way.

*Rule No. 3. The charlatan refuses to publish his data and/or respect the pre-established rules of validation and control. His theories always have the characteristic of being "difficult to reproduce" by others or cannot be disclosed. In general, he identifies the lack of 100% efficacy of official therapies or requests an impossible demonstration of them.*

Modern science comes into being when it moves away from pseudoscience and it does so with one of the key rules put forward by the father of the scientific method, Galileo Galilei: reproducibility. It is with this principle, for example, that chemistry disassociated itself from alchemy, in which concoctions prepared by wizards and swindlers were handed down in secret by esoteric sects of insiders. Repeatability, agreed rules and transparency: today these are the pilasters of scientific research. The charlatan always tries to avoid the rules of scientific validation, claiming exceptions from the experimental protocol, asking for secrecy or refusing permission to replicate the experiments in public and independent laboratories (naturally they are obliged to keep the invention confidential and the respect of intellectual property according to standard international rules). When these procedures and controls are obtained, and the results, obviously, prove the charlatan wrong, he claims failure to respect the "artisan" aspects of the experimentation or lays the blame on machines with different calibrations ignoring that, when they exist these aspects must be included in the details of the scientific protocol, so that each laboratory can be in a position to replicate the experiments—as is the case for all drugs and therapies validated today, without exception.

Aware of the weakness of his "cure", the charlatan tends to weaken the image of the rival official therapy. One classic strategy is to identify individual cases of failure or unexpected side effects in order to compare them with the failures of his own false therapy, knowing very well that the majority of patients do not have the instruments necessary for a correct evaluation of the risks/benefits ratio of a therapeutic treatment.

Another subtle rhetoric instrument to weaken the official therapy is the (manipulative) request for impossible proof: in the case of the vaccines, it is generally the request to conduct experiments on a wide population of children who have not been vaccinated in order to compare their neurocognitive and immunological parameters with those of vaccinated children. Today this request cannot be fulfilled, because no ethical committee would accept subjecting small human beings to the risk of fatal infections to prove alternative theories, moreover, without a scientific basis. As we have seen, however, what researchers have been able to do is to take the population data of the past and measure them against current ones, proving this way the importance of the vaccinations in improving the life expectancy of the immunized children as well as the absence of a greater rate of neurological and immunological pathologies. The request for impossible proof can also avail itself of an instrumental use of the temporal dimension: this takes place when the charlatan defers to a future time the appreciation of the proof of validity of his "cure". Released from the present and projected into the future, any false therapy whatsoever can enjoy credibility.

*Rule No. 4. The charlatan refuses to validate his theories through specialized literature. Rather, he uses the public square and the media where, as he is often a skilful communicator, he appeals to public opinion with guilt-inducing and emotionally engaging topics (terminally ill patients, children etc.).*

The only way to validate a scientific theory or a medical therapy is to submit it to so-called *peer review*, and subsequently to a body of control which, as anticipated several times, in the USA is the FDA and in Europe is the EMA and the individual national regulatory agencies. Today, more than ever, biomedical knowledge is fragmented into a series of disciplines and competences which do not always communicate with one another; therefore, only those who are experts in a specific disciplinary field can evaluate the efficacy of a product or therapeutic protocol. When a researcher believes he has found a promising line of therapeutic research, the first thing he does is look for confirmation among colleagues, nationally and internationally: he knows very well that science is a collective enterprise, where the success of the individual is only one stage allowed by the invaluable research of many others, and where self-certification is of no value. Every discovery becomes valid if shared and confirmed by competent colleagues and only when the public examination has been made, does it make sense to hold press conferences to disclose the information and seek international recognition. One of the typical features of the charlatan of false research is the so-called science by press conference, a definition which throws discredit on those scientists who organize them to publicize their discoveries before the scientific community has certified their reliability or even their innovativeness.

Just like the despotic and demagogical politician who avoids the democratic confrontation with his party colleagues or the institutions to establish "a direct contact with the people of the electorate", the charlatan avoids confrontation with the scientific community by directly intercepting the feelings of patients. Seeking public consent with emotionally engaging topics is a cognitive strategy which the charlatan uses to reduce the rational abilities of evaluation, in the hope that the "street" (and, therefore, politics, which depends on it through the vote) bends the regulatory agencies or providers of research funds to his needs. As in general he is an astute communicator, the charlatan knows very well that between an authority (possibly one of the greatest experts in the world on a specific therapy), who expresses doubts on the risks and benefits of a certain experimental protocol, and a couple of parents, who ask for "compassionate" treatment for their small child, terminally ill with a pathology for which there is no cure, the latter will also be the winners on the media level. This is a guilt-inducing strategy which uses the patient's body to obtain from politics, by overwhelming public pressure, the deregulation for the approval of drugs, in the name of a poorly understood notion of "compassionate treatment": it does not consist of (according to the vulgate in use today) the freedom of the patient to be treated at the expense of the state with unapproved therapies, in the name of a terminal clinical situation and the absence of available treatments. Compassionate treatment is something else, and it is also regulated, to protect patients. For a treatment to be compassionate, there have to be at least five parameters: it has to be applicable to a very limited number of patients, there already has to be an extensive file of solid scientific pre-clinical publications available, as well as a state of clinical experimentation of at least phase 1 (i.e. which insures it is not harmful), the company that manufactures the drug must promote its experimentation taking on the costs and without drawing economic advantage from it and lastly, the issue of the relative authorizations must take place under the close supervision of technical or regulatory bodies (FDA) in collaboration with clinical experts free of conflict of interest. Anything not according to these criteria is not medicine, but illegal activity advocated by charlatans.

When there is no therapy for a disease, the doctor is ethically obliged to reveal he is unable to offer treatment. Such an act of honesty and of respect towards the patient is not always perceived positively or accepted by a person in critical conditions. At the basis of choices that are "alternative" or "complementary" to traditional medicine, there are therefore despair, loneliness and the hope of patients and their families. Naturally, the rigorous and sincere doctor does not have less empathy for one patient than the doctor who wants to delude him; indeed, it is by working day after day in the laboratory, well out of the limelight and in the respect of the rules, sincerely admitting their errors, limits and successes, that biomedical researchers show patients their genuine compassion.

*Rule No. 5. The technique at which the charlatan is most skilful is perhaps the least evident one: he cuts out for himself the role of the misunderstood martyr.*

That of the misunderstood victim or opposed by the "system" is an excellent sociological and media strategy in which paradoxically, the charlatan, the more he is attacked, the more he benefits. Those who do not expose him give him an advantage, as they are accomplices in fostering the development of a fake therapy, but those who expose him also reinforce his social image, as he says he is a misunderstood victim who could cure thousands of patients, if only he were not prevented from this by a cynical and envious scientific community. The figure of the misunderstood martyr unexpectedly finds various social supports that can foster it. In the first place by catalysing the increasingly widespread social frustrations, all those who, today, especially because of the economic crisis, blame injustices of a political nature and obstacles of the institutional type on their failure to have reached satisfactory professional results (even only expected or imaginary). Secondly, the various interest groups which for years have been lobbying at political and economic level, for a deregulation of pharmacotherapies, also gain advantages from this figure. The length of time (more than 10 years), the countless control procedures and thousands of documents necessary before a drug can be put on to the market are all instruments used by the national public regulatory agencies to protect the health of citizens. Sometimes, these agencies are contrasted by the ambitions of private investors, who would like to obtain an economic return as soon as possible and not infrequently, they ride on the same demagogical claims as the charlatans to obtain a deregulation to their advantage. These two forces have recently been joined by a third one: what is known as the *Internet conspiracy theories*. The characteristics of the conspiracy theories present in the Internet, as mentioned in Chap. 1, go well with the figure of the charlatan who is a victim of the powers that be: blogs are full of narrations which describe powerful and rich political-economic lobbies which, in agreement with the corrupt state, plot against isolated figures of pure researchers who, as they are outside the games of power, fail to impose their revolutionary therapy.

The scientific enterprise shown as driven by victims and tormentors is, however, pure fiction, excellent for films, books and blogs, but not to understand reality. The scientist is a professional figure whose work is particularly subject to respecting rules and reciprocal control; this respect is perhaps present more strongly than in other categories, as he is at one and the same time both the legislator and the subject of the rules that he adopts, through a series of standard procedures such as the placebo effect, the double blind trial and the peer review.

# 5

# The Past, Present and Future of Vaccines

## The Evolutionary History of Naturally Acquired Immunity

When a mother gives birth to a child naturally, in addition to life and love, she gives her baby a third gift which is often ignored: immunity. When the baby passes through the vaginal canal, it comes into contact with a series of "good" bacteria that offer it the first form of adaptation to the surrounding environment. Selected by the adaptive dynamics that are established between the mother and her ecological niche—her relationship with the environment, food, infectious agents and various allergens—they colonize the intestinal tract of the baby, who will inherit a strain of bacteria that are already well adapted to the environment where it will live. Made up of 100 trillion cells with a gene pool that is 100 times greater than the human one, this set of bacteria, known as the *intestinal microbiome* (the bacterial flora)—today considered like a real organ—has essential functions for human health, such as exploiting the energy of components that are difficult to assimilate, producing useful vitamins, keeping the immune system efficient and above all, competing with pathogenic bacteria and defending us from the aggression of microorganisms. Recent studies have shown that children who are born by caesarean section develop in the first years of life, and often later as well, some complications linked to the malfunctioning of their immune system, not only because they do not have the beneficial maternal "contagion" of useful bacteria but also because they can be damaged by infections due to the pathogenic bacteria present on the skin and in the hospital environment (Dominguez-Bello et al. 2010). In particular, babies

© Springer International Publishing AG, part of Springer Nature 2018
A. Grignolio, *Vaccines: Are they Worth a Shot?*, https://doi.org/10.1007/978-3-319-68106-1_5

born by caesarean section have a greater rate of asthma, allergic reactions, anaphylactic shock (atopic syndromes) and colitic disorders (Gronlund et al. 1999; Salminen et al. 2004; Negele et al. 2004; Debley et al. 2005; Biasucci et al. 2008; Neu and Rushing 2011).

The colonization of the microbiome by every mother on her baby is, therefore, a sort of first natural vaccination of human beings, together with other mammals: an organism is exposed to an infectious agent that develops inside the body a series of reactions that protect it from future infections. In this case, however, the analogy has to be understood only in a general sense, as the mother's microbiome does not generate an infectious disease, and does not make the baby immune from future contacts with the bacteria transmitted, but generally reinforces the organism from aggression by pathogenic agents. The real form of "naturally acquired immunity" is, on the other hand, specific, as it is established between a given infectious agent and the host organism, which once the disease has been overcome, will remain immune. The adjective "natural" has to be emphasized here because vaccination is an artificial form of immunization which man has developed, inspired by the mechanisms that regulate the relations between *Homo sapiens* and germs in their reciprocal evolutionary history. However, before discussing the discovery of variolation, or of "artificially acquired immunity", by oriental cultures, a historical-evolutionary introduction has to be made.

The concept of pathocenosis, as already discussed, clearly explains that with the passage from nomad hunters-gatherers to members of a settled agricultural society, human beings underwent an important change in their nutritional and social habits. About 11,000 years ago, after the last glaciation, they went from small tribal structures of a few individuals, with limited offspring and scarce food, capable of covering several kilometres a day, to settled groups of increasingly numerous farmers who were organized in large urban settlements and social castes, with large supplies of food and lifestyles in close contact with animals, thanks to the discovery of the domestication of plants and species (birds, bovine and swine) suitable for breeding. The co-evolution between men and parasites also changed radically: whereas the hunters-gatherers had to coexist with (extracellular) infections caused by worms and parasites or by cutaneous excoriations but were not subject to epidemics—as the small size of the social groups and the isolation of the tribes prevented their propagation—the settled agricultural societies had to adapt to (intracellular) infections by viruses and bacteria which caused frequent epidemics, due both to the population density (which increased from 10 to 100 times with respect to the previous lifestyles), and to closely living with animals which began to transmit their infections to man (a phenomenon known as *zoonosis*). For example, think of measles which evolved from rinderpest or flu from pigs and birds and the fact that smallpox reached man from cattle or camels (or mice), whooping cough from pigs and dogs (the latter also transmit the fulminating virus of rabies), plague from rats, rabbits and hares and the devastating haemorrhagic fevers (including Ebola) from bats and monkeys—without considering all the infectious forms of which animals are, if not the origin, at least vectors: plague and typhus carried by rats, lie and ticks; tetanus and leishmaniasis by dogs; toxiplasmosis by cats; brucellosis by sheep and cattle; salmonellosis by farmyard animals such as chickens, pigs and cattle and by domestic reptiles such as tortoises and iguanas (Rezza 2010). All these diseases have been transmitted to man over thousands of years through blood, saliva, faeces and urine and have selected in our species some adaptive responses. In this evolutionary change, the parts of the organism that have undergone the greatest selective pressure have been the digestive tract and the immune system. This change of diet and a different relationship between carbohydrates and animal and plant proteins have altered the sources of the daily calorie intake, the metabolism, the enzyme apparatus and above all the intestinal microbiome and its dialogue with the immune system—a cross-talk which in turn has modified the inflammatory mediators and the immune competence cells in relation to the different type of infection (from extra- to intra-cellular) and the exposure time (from chronic to acute).

The immune system, after having adapted for thousands of years to fighting and living with chronic infections caused by parasitic microorganisms (protozoa) and worms (helminths, nemetodes), had to readapt to a new inflammatory context, made up of acute and contagious infections, which came in waves, caused by new enemies such as viruses, bacteria, microbacteria and fungi (Dobrovolskaya 2005; Wolfe et al. 2007; Kuipers et al. 2012; Rook et al. 2013).

In this, *Homo sapiens* has had to engage with the natural environment in a sort of reciprocal chase, a continuous and extenuating war between men and germs which has seen periods of balance (pathocenosis) alternate with sudden defeats (epidemics). These dynamics also explain the fortuitous primacy of Western cultures, i.e. how a casual bio-geographical context allowed the Caucasian populations of Eurasia to adapt to the evolutionary challenges better than other populations on the planet (such as the Chinese or the Sumerians) who in the first few thousands of years after the last glaciation were certainly not less developed. The human settlements that lived in the Euro-Asian plains were able to develop farming and the domestication of animals because nourishing plant species lived there (cereals, legumes and fruit trees), which could easily be cultivated thanks to the presence of water and temperate areas, as well as the many wild animals that were easy to tame and domesticate (cows, horses, sheep, goats and pigs), and useful both as food and to work in the fields and use as transport. In a large area, characterized by a uniform climate and without geographical barriers—unlike other continents such as Africa, the Americas and Oceania—domesticated animals and plants could be traded by the different populations through the trade routes, which helped facilitate the spread of the various farming techniques and technological innovations, as well as the development of the first units of measurement. Domestication meant not only plentiful food but also gaining (for the first time in the history of humanity and for several classes of society) large amounts of time, otherwise used for hunting and looking for sources of food. The discovery of writing emerged from the needs linked to storing and trading food and the regulation of the practices of worship. The organization of work allowed the formation of the working classes and of the nonproductive ones (such as the political and religious classes) which in time were organized into armies engaged in the conquest of adjacent territories. A central role in this evolution was played by artisans who in the Euro-Asian territories discovered deposits of materials (bronze, iron, steel) useful for forging weapons for defence and attack and who began to make spades, armour, carts and weapons of war while those assigned to military innovations domesticated horses for raids and plundering. These first forms of social organization produced a surplus of goods that led Euro-Asian civilizations to develop a flourishing trade which over the centuries shifted to the Mediterranean basin to produce ships for sea transport, weapons for the conquest of lands and goods and metal utensils to modify nature and the surrounding environment. The Caucasian populations drew enormous benefits from these fortuitous events: their social organization, the techniques for growing, storing and transporting food and the use of steel instruments and efficient weapons dominated the resistance of the populations they confronted for the whole of the prehistoric period and over the last three thousands of years, these advantages have been inherited by the European cultures which originated from those populations (Diamond 1998).

Of the many advantages, however, perhaps it was the least obvious one that favoured the European populations: the cyclical spread of epidemics due to animal domestication. The leap of species that viruses and bacteria from animals regularly make, infecting man, allowed the European population to develop a very important co-evolutionary adaptation: thanks to a costly natural selection, this population has acquired a form of immunization and adaptation to germs which has allowed on the one hand the survival of the immunolog- ically most resistant individuals (who have transmitted this characteristic to their descendants) and on the other the survival of the infectious agents which have attenuated their virulence to be able to spread without the risk of annihilating their host (and therefore becoming extinct). In addition to armour made from resistant alloys, the Europeans who set off to conquer other continents unconsciously also had the advantage of an internal armour, the immunological one. Their immune system was better equipped to face a broad spectrum of infectious diseases with which other populations had never come into contact—which exposed the latter to devastating epidemics. Of course, in the European populations as well, the various outbreaks of epidemics decided and deviated human destiny, also influencing the outcome of the great territorial conquests or wiping out entire urban settlements.

The first documented plague to have influenced the course of Western history—as well as the first case of a relationship between history and medicine—was the plague of Athens in 430 BC during the Peloponnesian War. The outcome is known: after a first success by the Athenian army led by the valorous strategist Pericles, a terrible epidemic broke out in the Attic city (overpopulated and with promiscuous hygiene and health conditions), probably of typhus—or possibly a form of haemorrhagic fever—which weakened its inhabitants and killed Pericles himself, allowing the victory of Sparta. This event, with the subsequent defeat of the second expedition to Sicily, marked the definitive military and political decline of Athens, the cradle of Western democracy. As mentioned, the historian who provided the details of this epidemic, the first known to us, was Thucydides: in his writings, the phenomenon of natural immunization from infectious diseases was described for the first time, when he stated that those who recover "are now safe" because on "you do not fall a second time into the illness, or at least a possible relapse does to lead to death." It clearly emerges from the words of the Greek historian that immunity is a "specific" phenomenon because it is valid only for the infectious disease that infected the survivor, "acquired" naturally due to the infection and that it is a phenomenon that is "remembered" by the organism because subsequent exposures to the pathogenic agent do not cause infection or cause it in mild forms only. The purpose of Thucydides' meticulous description consisted of offering all the details of a traumatic historical event, in order to be able to recognize similar phenomena in the case they appeared again in the future: a prophylactic or educational use of history.

In the same region and in the same years, curiously, there was another significant fact in the relationship between history and medicine: medicine came into being, thanks to Hippocrates (460–370 circa BC), as did history thanks to Herodotus (484–430 circa BC), two disciplines which found a common theoretical ground around the word *historia*, which came from medical language and indicated the act of examining and putting together different cases and situations to try and discover their natural common causes (Momigliano 1985). From the very origins then, medicine and history share some methodological characteristics in their diagnosis of reality, based on extrapolations from a series of signs and symptoms.

In addition to the plague of Athens, there was another great historical event in which infections played a crucial role. We have to jump about 2000 years ahead and change continent to go to the times of the conquest of Mexico by Hernán Cortés (1485–1547), the Spanish condottiere who, in 1519, with only 500 men, was able to annihilate the far more impressive army and Aztec empire ruled over by Montezuma. It was not the weapons or the military training of the Spanish army that had the better of the Aztecs, but rather an infection of smallpox that the Conquistadores brought with them from Europe and which was unknown to the immune system of the American indigenous peoples. In the early sixteenth century, the population of Mexico was made up of some 25 million people, which the infectious epidemics brought by the Europeans reduced by 98% in only 100 years—a hecatomb of 22 million deaths—declining to only 700,000 inhabitants in 1623. The Europeans were more resistant to the infections than the indigenous populations because, having been isolated from Europe since the times of the last glaciation (when they could use the Bering Strait), they did not enjoy the evolutionary benefits due to the natural selection by epidemics as an indirect phenomenon of domestication. The indigenous peoples of the New World were naturally adapted to the infectious diseases in their own environment, for example syphilis—the only disease, basically chronic and not fatal, that they passed on to the Europeans—but on the immunological level they were not covered by the variety of infectious agents to which the Europeans had been used for thousands of years.

Before, during and after the plague of Athens and the epidemic of Cortés, there were naturally countless plagues that decimated the world population. The death of the Pharaoh Ramses V in 1157 BC was caused by smallpox, as well shown by the signs which can still be seem on the mummy's face, and polio was also common amongst the ancient Egyptians, as testified by a stele of the XVIII dynasty (1403–1365 BC) showing a victim with his right leg impaired by the infectious disease. In the vulgar era, the various outbreaks of epidemics of plague, smallpox, measles and flu decreased the European population, causing the deaths of over one billion individuals: these pandemics include, in 167 AD in Rome, the outbreak of what is known as the *Antonine plague* (smallpox or measles, brought back by the legionnaires from Mesopotamia) in which 30,000 men died; what was known as the *bubonic plague* or *Justinian plague* (from Constantinople and the Red Sea) which reached Rome in 543 killing 40% of the population and at least 25 million all over the world in the 20 waves of epidemics which followed until 767; and the return of the bubonic plague, called the *black plague*, which struck Europe in the middle of the fourteenth century and left a third of the continent's population dead, i.e. between 50 and 70 million people. From the sixteenth century onwards, a number of pandemics of flu are clearly described: four in the sixteenth century, five in the seventeenth century and two in the nineteenth century (in 1830 and in 1890), until the hecatomb already mentioned caused by *Spanish flu* which caused between 50 and 100 million deaths in the years following the First World War.

## Artificially Acquired Immunity: The Success and Safety of Vaccines

The first contagious disease in history that man tried to control through acquired immunity was smallpox, around the beginning of the year 1000 AD. It took 800 years before the principles that had allowed the oriental populations to intuit the mechanism underlying the attenuation and immunization from smallpox could be applied to other infectious diseases: in between, there were millions of deaths.

The roots of immunity are remote and are confused with magic thought. As seen in Chap. 2, a concept that this archaic form of thought has often shared with prescientific medicine lies in the idea that "like cures like" according to the laws of analogy and empathy that regulate the relations between the elements, their forces and the energies of the world, both in the microcosm and in the macrocosm. In the absence of a physiological explanation, prescientific man of various eras and latitudes tried to treat human disorders by imagining simple mechanisms of the balance of the natural elements (air, earth, water, fire), governed by forces of attraction and repulsion, beneficial and malefic, curative and poisonous effects, conditioned by astral or divine influences, according to a trend in accordance with the alternation of the seasons, which concealed a plan of pre-established and finalistic development. In this conceptual framework, healers and shamans offered their patients herbs, decoctions and antidotes which, depending on the cases, had the aim of balancing the effects of the disease or exacerbating them until their strength was exhausted.

The cultures of Asia Minor in the Anatolian peninsula of the first century BC had elaborated these concepts in a fairly advanced way, theorizing what today we call *Mithridatism*, the idea that it is possible to artificially acquire immunity to poisons by being gradually exposed to them, and *hormesis*, the principle according to which small doses of toxic substances become innocuous or beneficial—a principle already exploited by various animals, including primates, with the use of psychotropic plants and fermented fruit (Dudley 2000). It was like this for Mithridates VI (111-63 BC), king of Pontus (present-day Turkey) who, fearing a conspiracy, asked the court physician to prepare antidotes against poisons. Legend has it that the gradual exposure to the toxins did not affect the health of the sovereign at all, who lived a long life, and, when he was defeated by Pompey Magnus, to take his own life he had to stab himself as every poison was ineffective. Many other ancient cultures, for example African ones, have popular traditions according to which it is possible for men and animals to develop immunity to the poison of snakes through gradual exposure.

Some sources date the first forms of artificial immunization through variolation, the exposure to infected human material, to China in the second century AD, during the Han and Jin dynasties, others to the year 1000 AD during the Sung dynasty (920–1279). Without any doubt, the practice of blowing into the nostrils of healthy people the dust of crusts extracted from individuals affected by attenuated forms of smallpox, for prophylactic purposes, was widespread in China between the end of the eighteenth and the start of the nineteenth centuries (La Condamine 1773; Ma 1995; Xie and Zhang 2000; Xin-Zhong 2003; Buck 2003; Flower 2008; Needham et al. 2010). Other historical sources trace similar procedures back to India and Africa, although with different grafting mechanisms: using small lances covered with smallpox pus to be inserted subcutaneously (inoculation) or by wrapping healthy people in infected sheets (Davis 1978; Greenough 1980; Moulin 1996; Gross and Sepkowitz 1998; Brimnes 2004; Dinc and Ulman 2007). However, one other exception in the treatment of smallpox must be noted, with respect to other contagious diseases: for leprosy, measles, plague and flu the various human communities worked out only forms of postinfectious containments linked to hygiene and health procedures aimed at isolating the infected patient (think of quarantine and lazarettos), for smallpox forms of prevention and the greatest proximity with the infectious agent, such as inoculation or exposure to the virus, were used. It was, therefore, with smallpox that active prevention emerged, through the idea that it is possible to be "artificially" immunized, acquiring protection against the effects of the disease contracted naturally. It is an empirical procedure to which the populations were subjected, with fluctuating resistances, after having noted how this way mortality was significantly reduced, going from about 30% to a mortality of 2.3%.

These procedures arrived in the countries bordering Europe from Asia to the Middle East via the Silk Road, in the seventeenth century: the inhabitants of the Caucasus inoculated the virus of smallpox in women for the notables of the Ottoman Empire, the famous Circassian slaves, to avoid them being disfigured. Inoculation then spread to Greece, Thessaly and Turkey, from where it was imported to Europe. The first time that the West heard of variolation was through the publications of the British Royal Society, thanks to the letters of two Italian doctors from the university of Padua, based in Constantinople: that of 1714 (but referred to 1713) by Emanuele Timone (1669–1720), dragoman of Genoese origin at the service of the Embassy of Great Britain, and that of 1715 (published in 1716) by Jacopo Pilarino (1659–1718), originally from Cefalonia, the Venetian consul at the Sublime Port of Constantinople. The communications were picked up by doctors and intellectuals like James Woodward in 1714 and James Jurin in 1718 in England and by Louis Duvrac in 1723 in France, up to being discussed in the important Parisian salons by Voltaire, who dedicated the eleventh of his *Letters on the English* (1742) to vaccination and Charles-Marie de La Condamine, who even wrote a whole work on the topic, *Mémoire sur l'inoculation de la petite vérole* (1754).

The circulation of these writings and the debate that developed in Europe between supporters and detractors of variolation would never have been possible without the example, in 1720, of Lady Mary Wortley Montagu (1689–1762), the aristocratic wife of the British consul to Constantinople: disfigured in her youth by smallpox, she decided to have her eldest son variolated at the Ottoman court. Thanks to the promotion of Lady Montagu in England, in 1721, the practice was experimented on prisoners and orphaned children and the next year on the two sons of Princess Caroline von Brandenburg; from then on, it spread through the aristocracy and the ruling families in Europe which devoured its wider adoption by the population. In Europe, the practice of variolation which circulated was that of *arm to arm*, which consisted of organizing public meetings in which patients with tenuous forms of smallpox, in a certain period of the infectious cycle, would offer their pustules to healthy people who, infected through a surface scarification on the shoulder, during the subsequent meetings could (voluntarily or against payment) in turn offer themselves as new immunizers; this practice was naturally risky from a hygienic point of view, because at times, together with smallpox many other diseases were transmitted, especially venereal ones.

The fundamental stage in the evolution of artificially acquired immunity came, as seen in Chap. 2, thanks to the work of Edward Jenner, although he was not the first to discover vaccination—considering that the primacy goes to at least six figures, including the English farmer Benjamin Jesty (1737–1816), who between 1774 and 1789 used it empirically on his own family, the surgeon and pharmacist (known to Jenner) John Fewster (1738–1824), who ran a business for the promotion of variolation, and the German teacher Peter Plett (1766–1823), who was, however, the first to scientifically prove that this practice was more effective and practical than variolation (Hammarsten et al. 1979; Gross and Sepkowitz 1998; Pead 2003; Plett 2006; Thurston and Williams 2015). Jenner, who during his adolescence was inoculated with smallpox, in the years of his medical training worked in the countryside, where farmers lived in close contact with their animals and their diseases. Like Jetsy and Fewster, he also realized, inspired by popular tales and his experience as a variolating doctor, that the people who milked cows did not contract smallpox—easily recognizable because without signs on the face of the disease, as well as being useful social figures for the support of persons infected during epidemics—because they were protected by a previous infection of cowpox, a milder form than smallpox as shown by the slight cutaneous breakouts that the milkers contracted on contact with the excoriations present on the udders of the cows. Jenner wanted to study these experiences further and after several studies, decided to conduct an experiment which turned out to be revolutionary: in 1796 he obtained from the pustules of Sarah Nelmes, a local milkmaid who had contracted cowpox, an extract of pus which he inoculated (vaccination) into an 8-year-old boy, James Phipps, who developed a mild form of smallpox and was subsequently exposed to smallpox (variolation), being immune to it. Jenner proved that the aggressive natural human variety of smallpox had not developed an infection because the boy had been immunized by the naturally attenuated variety of cowpox. In a note sent to the *Royal Society* in 1798, he scientifically proved that it was more effective and safer to immunize human beings by infecting them with cowpox—a practice defined *vaccination*—rather than using pustules of smallpox. The cowpox had preferable side effects compared to smallpox, because the passage of the relative pus, as well as containing a less aggressive virus (and therefore less risky), prevented the transmission of other then common human venereal diseases such as syphilis, hepatitis B and tuberculosis. Furthermore, unlike human beings, the cows could be put in a serial culture to produce large amounts of vaccinal matter, useful in the periods of epidemics, to be collected, purified and stored. They could also be easily transported to villages and could offer the vaccine for prophylactic purposes even in the periods when the human epidemic had ended. In a short time, the practice of Jenner's vaccination spread from England to the rest of the continent.

The last step before industrial production of vaccines was owed to the French chemist and microbiologist Louis Pasteur (1822–1895), who between 1879 and 1885 showed the possibility of artificially attenuating the virulence of other agents pathogenic for man, such as anthrax (1881) and rabies (1885), on the model of the anti-smallpox vaccine. He also understood the social and economic importance of veterinary vaccination, developing the vaccinations against fowl cholera and anthrax for cattle, horses and sheep. The method used by Pasteur had four phases: isolating the pathogenic agents, cultivating them, trying to attenuate the infectious cultures obtained (e.g. by exposing them to sources of heat or letting them decant for a long time) and lastly, injecting them into animals, to cause mild infections and subsequent immunity. This series of fundamental conceptual passages (isolation, cultivation, attenuation, injection) laid down the bases for vaccinology and immunology. Even though it would take another 60 years before understanding the mechanism with which the organism actively produces adaptive antibodies to fight newer and newer infectious agents—in 1957, thanks to the Australian Nobel Prize winning virologist, Frank Macfarlane Burnet (Tauber and Podolsky 1997) (1899–1985)—at the end of the nineteenth century, Pasteur had grasped that it was an active mechanism, i.e. something that was produced by the organism after the injection of the attenuated infectious serum, which protected the host, making it immune to subsequent exposures. Pasteur's discovery fitted into a new phase of biomedical thought in which, thanks to his contributions and those of the German doctor and microbiologist Robert Koch (1843–1910), the theory of the microbial origin of infections was outlined. They had understood how infectious diseases are caused by pathogenic agents which, similarly to a parasite, enter the host organism, infecting it and duplicating itself, to then spread in the surrounding population through body fluids, saliva, blood and dejections.

From Pasteur onwards, the race towards the production of vaccines was impressive, at the rate of almost three new vaccines every decade.

Passive immunity was also discovered in the same period, thanks to the production of antibodies generated by animals and then transferred to man, who therefore becomes immune not due to active production but to passive reception of antibodies. Various antibacterial serums were then prepared—against dysentery, gonococcus, meningococcus, the plague, staphylococcus, streptococcus and typhus—obtained by immunizing animals (horses, cattle, sheep and rabbits) in quantities such as to be able to be stored and sold. This was how the season of serotherapy was inaugurated, with the early years spent in an attempt to purify animal serums, to avoid allergic reactions in man. There is more. In close competition with his French colleagues Jules Héricourt (1850–1938) and Charles Richet (1850–1935), who described the principles of serotherapy in 1888, and even tried to use the antibodies present in the serum for a cure for cancer (1895), in 1890 in Germany Emil von Behring (1854–1917) and Shibasaburo Kitasato (1852–1931) discovered the diphtheria antitoxin serum. The pair proved that the bacteria which causes diphtheria is in itself harmless, but produces highly harmful toxins which can be fought by antibodies, and that these can be produced by an animal, extracted from its serum (immune serum) and, lastly, injected in purified form (toxoids) into man, giving him immunity. Behring, therefore, proved that the immunity acquired with a serum produced by other organisms—a major conceptual revolution—can be transferred and Kitasato used the same mechanism to produce the tetanus antitoxin serum.

It is difficult to understand today just how important Behring's discovery of the diphtheria antitoxin was, which is why it is important to tell a famous story which has now been forgotten. In Central Park, there is a curious metal statue of a dog, but unfortunately its plaque is ignored by the many parents and children who visit the splendid green lung of New York at the weekend. The dog in the sculpture is Balto and its story is the heroic phase, once socially recognized, of vaccinations, of which today all trace has unfortunately been lost. In mid-December 1924 in Nome, a village of 10,000 souls on the eastern Alaska coast looking on to the Bering Strait, where the territory of the United States borders with Russia, the village doctor, Curtis Welch, started to notice in the infantile population a worrying increase of tonsillitis which after a few days turned out to be an incipient epidemic of diphtheria. Things quickly got dramatically worse: in a month, five children died from suffocation due to the toxins of the bacterium. Welch discovered that the doses of anti-diphtheria serum in the village had expired and in any case were insufficient and the winter months made transport by sea or air impossible. The only chance to save the whole village, now in quarantine, was put in a telegram in which Washington was asked to send immediately a million doses of serum—which passively transferred immunity because it already contained the antibodies against the toxins; after a few years it was possible to detoxify the toxins creating injectable toxoids, a safer and longer lasting procedure because it was capable of creating active immunity, as is the case today when part of the trivalent diphtheria–tetanus–pertussis vaccine is produced. A crisis cell met which voted on what seemed to be the only solution: to organize a relay of sledge dogs, but the distance that separated Nome from Nenana, the only accessible point of departure of the serum, was 1085 km and the trip usually took 25 days. This was too long. The best racing and transport teams were, thus, recruited for a total of 20 men and 150 dogs which were able to cover the distance in 5 days and 7 hours, at temperatures that plunged to 40° below zero. The radio and newspapers of the time followed the event with great public enthusiasm, so much so that the dog that made the last stretch, Balto, leapt to front page news—even though the hardest part of the route had been one by another dog, Togo. In the following months, a short film and the New York statue were dedicated to Balto. The consequence of this media success was that the anti-diphtheria coverage in the US population recorded an unprecedented increase. In Alaska, a race for sledge dogs is still held every year in Iditarod to commemorate the event. The story of Balto with the cold and isolated places well relates the paradox of modern societies towards vaccinations, where it is comfort, education and a high social level that creates the doubts about the vaccines.

In the years following the discoveries by von Behring and Kitasato, the antiserums against the toxins of snake poison were produced, offering a pocket preparation (with vial and syringe) useful for men and animals living in infested areas. The refinement of the knowledge of the highly specific relationships between antibodies and toxins or between antibodies and the reactive parts (antigenic) of the pathogenic agents also allowed the development of serology and serodiagnostics. These are the technologies which by putting into a common solution blood samples extracted from patients and some specific reagents, biochemical reactions of recognition can be obtained and the presence in the blood of specific diseases can be identified—as in the case of the Wasserman or reaction test for syphilis—offering for the first time fairly reliable diagnoses, useful in particular for different diseases that had similar exanthematic or clinical manifestations.

Serotherapy, with its ability to obtain antibodies from survivors of infectious diseases for which there are not yet any vaccines, is still today a valid therapeutic instrument, as shown by its wide use in the recent Ebola epidemic (where the affected people were given antibodies of survivors). Serotherapy which can, therefore, be seen as a passive and therapeutic form of vaccination—which is, as has been seen, active and preventive—is also at the basis of one of the most important therapeutic discoveries in recent years: the monoclonal antibodies of animal or human origin, produced in laboratories and with an absolute specificity of reaction, are very effective in blocking some proteins or metabolic pathways which favour the development of cancer or in reactivating biochemical processes damaged by autoimmune diseases and aspire treating some neurodegenerative diseases such as Alzheimer's disease, Huntington's disease and multiple sclerosis (Mazumdar 1995; Watier 2009;

Daguet and Watier 2011, 2012; Panza et al. 2014; Todd et al. 2014; Lorefice et al. 2014).

Going back to vaccines, others came after Pasteur's against the virus of rabies, discovered in 1885: the following year for cholera and typhus; in 1897 for the plague; in 1923 for diphtheria; in 1926–1927 for pertussis, tetanus and tuberculosis; in 1935 for yellow fever; in 1955 for polio; between 1963 and 1969 for measles, mumps and rubella; and in the following years those against meningitis (various strains in 1975, 1985, 2013), pneumonia (1977), hepatitis B and A (1981, 1995), chicken pox (1995), *Papilloma virus* (2006) and many others for minor diseases (Plotkin and Plotkin 2011). This was an exciting race that man was winning against contagious diseases, after millions of deaths and indescribable suffering. Let's have a look at their main stages, to understand the various categories of vaccines, to then conclude with the mechanisms which certify their safety.

In 1921, the doctor and bacteriologist Albert Calmette (1863–1933) and the veterinary surgeon Camille Guérin (1872–1961), French researchers at the Pasteur Institute in Lille, produced the first vaccine against tuberculosis (TBC), a disease which generates meningitis and lung diseases, caused by a redoubtable microbacterium (*Mycobacterium tuberculosis*).

Leprosy is also caused by a deadly microbacterium (*Mycobacterium leprae*), of which the prefix myco- must not suggest a fungal nature, but only to a geometry of growth similar to that typical of fungi. Based on the Jenner and Pasteur models, Calmette and Guérin attempted to use the cow form of tuberculosis (*Mycobacterium bovis*) discovering that, unlike with smallpox, it was not at all attenuated and often led to the death of the patient who was inoculated with it. They then found themselves faced with the problem of keeping the bacterium alive—to allow the organism to have an antibody response and, therefore, the subsequent immunity—at the same time attenuating its virulence. After various attempts, they realized that a culture medium based on potato, glycerine and bile tended to attenuate the pathogenicity of the bacterium, but many cultures and generations were necessary, over no less than 13 years (1908–1921), to obtain the so-called *Bacillus Calmette Guérin* (BCG), an attenuated living microorganism coming from bacteria of bovine tuberculosis, which could be used as a vaccine against human tuberculosis. Today, it is the vaccine that is most widely used in the world. Its diffusion started with the International Campaign for tuberculosis which, launched after the Second World War, in about 3 years vaccinated 8 million children and almost 14 million people, especially in Eastern Europe. Before the diffusion of BCG, it is estimated that tuberculosis had mowed down, in 200 years, a billion people, including, as is well known, several generations of artists, intellectuals and writers (like Pascal, Spinoza, Chopin, Kafka, Molière, Gramsci, Modigliani and Eleanor Roosevelt). Today, it is administered to more than eighty million children, and it is effective above all to prevent tubercular meningitis and military tuberculosis, while it is less effective against pulmonary tuberculosis. Today. this still affects one-third of humanity (two billion people) at the rate of 1,25,000 infections a day. These figures explain better than any argument why, in the case of one of the most effective vaccines ever, like BCG, it is absolutely necessary to continue developing and improving vaccines (Mantovani and Florianello 2016, p. 48).

The era of the development of vaccines started when, in 1937, the South African doctor Max Theiler (1899–1972) developed the vaccine against yellow fever, caused by a virus which infects man and some primates using mosquitoes as vectors. In the mid-1930s, he discovered that embryonated chicken eggs—fertilized and used at a certain stage of development of the embryo of the chick—represent an efficient, practical and cheap culture medium for the growth of the virus: thanks to these, the viruses of flu and yellow fever could be cultivated and the relative vaccines produced. It took Theiler several years to obtain the vaccine and during this time he attenuated the virus, passing it through more than a 100 cultures, using mice; once he had obtained the attenuated form he injected it into Rhesus macaques, immunizing them. Attenuation through the passages of culture of particularly aggressive infectious or toxic agents represented a serious time hurdle and economic obstacle in the race towards the production of vaccines. The problem was solved by the French veterinary surgeon Gaston Ramon (1886–1963) who, from the 1920s, discovered that formaldehyde (which was talked about in Chap. 3) could attenuate the dangerousness of the toxin of tetanus and diphtheria. This method, still used today, together with the production of adjuvants (also discovered by Ramon) made the production of vaccines fast, safe and effective. The vaccines with living and attenuated pathogenic agents are, for example, those against measles, mumps and rubella (MMR); chicken pox; flu (the nasal spray); rotavirus; herpes zoster (or shingles); yellow fever; and, as we will see, one of the two vaccines against polio (the Salk vaccine administered orally).

In 1948, the combined (trivalent) vaccine for diphtheria, tetanus and pertussis (DTP) made its appearance: put on to the US market for the first time in 1948, it was obtained from the combination of a vaccine created in the 1920s containing the inactivated bacillus of pertussis, with inactivated toxins (toxoids) of diphtheria and tetanus produced in the 1930s thanks to the Ramon method. In 1981, an acellular version was developed, used from the 1990s onwards, which drastically reduced the adverse reactions. Vaccines are evolving all the time, but, as mentioned several times, this is completely useless if the quota necessary for herd cover is not reached. The pathogens contained in this combined trivalent vaccine are very aggressive, contagious and with significant mortality rates. Let's have a look at them.

Death caused by the virus of diphtheria (*Corynebacterium diphtheriae*), which often affects children, occurs by suffocation caused by an abnormal swelling of the throat (diphtheric croup). Today diphtheria "is still endemic in many developing countries, while, thanks to the diffusion of the vaccination, the last case of the disease in the paediatric age group in Italy was in 1995" (Mantovani and Florianello 2016, p. 41), but the bacterium has not disappeared and is very present amongst us, as the cases, previously discussed, of the epidemic in the states of the former Soviet Union in the 1990s and the more recent ones in Spain show. The same applies for tetanus and pertussis. The vaccine for tetanus needs various booster doses and while its diffusion is close to the safety threshold in the paediatric population of advanced countries, in Africa and Asia it still continues to claim many victims (from 30% to 50% of the cases of infection, especially in babies). Death caused by tetanus is particularly dramatic, through a spastic paralysis which affects the neck and face (the latter contracts, assuming an unnerving grin, known as the "sardonic smile") to then spread to the thorax and the abdomen and lastly contracting the limbs and the whole body arches tensely. Pertussis, on the other hand, is one of the most contagious infectious diseases, which in Italy until the 1990s counted more than 13,000 cases a year: today the WHO estimates that in the world there are between 20 and 50 million cases with 3,00,000 deaths—even in Europe, where deaths are one in every 1,00,000 cases (Mantovani and Florianello 2016, p. 42).

The new conquests in the fight against polio also opened up new scenarios in the production of vaccines. In this process, the invention and development of techniques of cultivating tissues (specifically monkey's kidneys) was essential. It allowed replicating the virus of polio up to attenuating or killing it. This procedure revealed that the polio virus, although it had been killed (or inactivated), was still able to create an immune reaction. The efficacy for the purposes of immunization of the killed pathogenic agents represents an innovation, because it proved how, in some cases (e.g. in hepatitis, in rabies and in the Salk vaccine against polio), the immune system succeeds nevertheless in producing antibodies and immunity without any risk of reactivating the infectious agent. The origin of the victory of science against this dreaded virus is to be sought in the National Foundation for Infantile Paralysis—established in 1938 by Franklin Delano Roosevelt, who believed he had been paralyzed by polio—and in the *March of Dimes*, which collected huge amounts of funding to help polio patients and support the search for a vaccine. The vaccines that defeated polio were developed by Jonas Salk, who in 1953 created a killed vaccine (administered with a subcutaneous injection), and Albert Sabin, who in 1955 obtained an attenuated one (administered orally). The Sabin vaccine was more effective when the cases are numerous: in a few decades polio was eradicated from developed countries and today only religious and tribal prejudices oppose the vaccination campaigns (as in Afghanistan, Nigeria, Pakistan and recently Syria) that prevent achieving global eradication.

During the 1960s, vaccines against measles, mumps and rubella were developed. As already mentioned in Chap. 1, the leading figure in vaccinology after the Second World War was the American microbiologist Maurice Hilleman (1919–2005), who worked on the vaccine against measles, created nine of the vaccines most used today (including those against mumps, rubella, hepatitis A, hepatitis B and pneumonia) and in 1971 developed the second most important combined vaccine after DTP, the trivalent measles–mumps–rubella (MMR). Hilleman is rightly considered "the most important vaccinologist in history" (Robert Gallo, in Maugh 2005) and he is perhaps the man who in history has saved most lives: about eight million a year, according to an estimate published in "Nature" (Dove 2005).

Towards the end of the 1970s, the cases of natural infection of smallpox (*Variola minor*) were very rare and in 1976 the last case was recorded in Africa with the infection of Ali Maow Maalin, the cook in a Somali hospital who became famous as the last individual in the history of humanity to have contracted one of the most feared natural scourges of all times; 3 years later, in Geneva, the WHO officially certified the eradication of smallpox from the globe.

1981 was the year of the first vaccine against hepatitis B (obtained by extracting antibodies form the blood of patients, whilst today more effective and safer versions are available, based on techniques of DNA manipulation), the virus which is responsible for a chronic disease which can lead to the onset of liver tumours; therefore, this vaccine is effectively the first one that is preventive against oncological diseases (the second, we will see, is the one against *Papilloma virus*). Introduced into Italy in 1991, it has been capable of reducing infections by 80%.

The last stage of the "classic" vaccines is represented by the development, between 1985 and 1987, by four American researchers, including David H. Smith (1932–1999), of the first conjugate vaccine against the *Haemophilus influenzae* of type b bacterium (Hib). This bacterium causes meningitis and other children's diseases and is covered by a capsule of complex sugars (polysaccharides, the same ones that cover the pneumococcus and meningococcus, which is why conjugate vaccines will also be produced against these bacteria) which lets it elude the view of the immune system, a strategy which researchers have got round by conjugating the polysaccharide with a protein, in order to make it reactive and visible, and give it immunogenicity—i.e. the ability to trigger the immune response and remember the polysaccharide as antigens.

Lastly, between 2006 and 2009, the vaccine against the *Papilloma virus* (HPV) was produced. This virus is responsible every year for 250,000 deaths and 400,000 new cases of uterine cancer which, together with breast cancer, is the commonest female tumour. An erroneous popularization describes it as ineffective and of exclusive interest for the female gender (it is recommended to 12-year olds before the start of sexual activity), forgetting that it is also transmitted by sexual intercourse to men, in whom it can generate a neoplasia in the head and neck (Mantovani and Florianello 2016, p. 46). In Western countries, the vaccine is spreading gradually and with some resistance (due mainly to disinterest or lack of information) even though the U.S. National Institute of Cancer estimates that it can reduce the number of deaths from cervical cancer by two-thirds.[1]

Some data on the risks are now required, even though we know that figures are "cold data" without any persuasive capacity. Today, thanks to the use of vaccines, the cases of diphtheria, measles, rubella, mumps, pertussis, tetanus and diseases caused by *Haemophilus influenzae* have been reduced by 98%, which shows how they are the most effective drugs in the world, by far exceeding those in the second place—drugs against rheumatic fever and rheumatic heart disease, which reach an efficacy of "only" 75% (Rappuoli and Vozza 2009, p. 36). The good news is finished. In the twentieth century, almost 1.7 billion people died from infectious diseases. Here are some of the more dramatic figures: 400 million deaths from smallpox, 96.7 million deaths from measles, 38.1 million deaths from pertussis, more than 37 million deaths from tetanus, 12.7 million deaths from hepatitis B and almost 22 million deaths from meningitis.[2] In particular, in the Western world, mass vaccinations have allowed avoiding the deaths of 500 million people (just under the current total population of the 28 countries of the EU in 2014) and in the future, i.e. in the decade from 2011 to 2020, they will allow avoiding the death

---

[1] National Institutes of Health, National Cancer Institute, Human Papillomavirus (HPV) Vaccines. Why Are These Vaccines Important? http://tinyurl.com/ouxokgn
[2] WHO Global Burden of Disease, WHO Mortality Report, "British Medical Journal", commissioned by the Wellcome Collection Nov 2012 "Twentieth Century Death", http://tinyurl.com/lrwk5po; data http://bit.ly/20thdeath; image: http://tinyurl.com/cwq65uo

of 25 million people, or 2.5 million people a year, 7000 a day, 300 every hour, 5 every minute.[3]

In conclusion, it has to be remarked that the fear over the safety of vaccines is not a real problem, in the sense that although it has a place in social fears, it is non-existent in the medical-scientific community—except the very rare cases (0.02 and 0.04%, respectively, in the USA and in Italy) which have been mentioned. These fears, however, have had a positive result: they have allowed the scientific community to extend an unprecedented network of world control. The safety of vaccines is proven by global epidemiological data, monitored and updated on a weekly basis, and evaluated by third-party and independent international bodies, which recruit the members of the evaluation committee on the basis of great competence and absence of conflict of interests—in order to avoid any of them being an affiliate of companies that produce the vaccine which is being evaluated. Two important and independent control bodies fulfil this delicate task, one European and one American. Let's start with the latter.

The VAERS (Vaccine Adverse Event Reporting System) is a national programme to monitor the safety of vaccines co-sponsored by the Centers for Disease Control and Prevention (CDC)—which, since 1990, has used an extensive network of electronic data shared on the Internet, the *Vaccine Safety Datalink* (VSD)[4]—and the FDA, the main national institution of public health in the United States. The VAERS is a programme of post-marketing monitoring which collects information on adverse reactions or unwanted events which take place after the administration of vaccines, and was created in 1990 following a law of 1986, which required healthcare operators and manufacturers of vaccines to report to the U.S. Department of Health the specific adverse events after the administration of recommended and routine vaccines. This programme receives about 30,000 reports per year and about 89–90% of the reports describe mild adverse events, such as a temperature, local reactions and episodes of crying or irritability; the remaining reports reflect more severe adverse events which involve hospitalization, temporary or permanent invalidity up to rare cases of risk of life and at times deaths—which, it has to be noticed, appear out of tens of millions of administrations to the US population, amounting to about 320 million inhabitants. Any parent, relation or acquaintance can send the communication of unwanted effects from a vaccine to VAERS but the site clearly states that false or untruthful

---

[3] Data based on WHO, Decade of Vaccines. Global Vaccine Action Plan 2011–2020: http://tinyurl.com/zjdvf67
[4] Vaccine Safety Datalink (VSD), http://tinyurl.com/oyknvz4

communications on health issues are punishable by fines and imprisonment. The structure of VAERS was designed to perform some key functions, including: to record new, unusual or rare adverse events (VAEs, *Vaccines Adverse Events*); to monitor in real time the increase of such events; to identify the potential risk factors of the patient for particular types of adverse events; to identify possible defective batches of vaccine; to carefully evaluate the safety of newly licensed vaccines. VAERS has proven to be very effective in identifying flaws in the vaccinal system, promptly providing the scientific and institutional community with reports of possible adverse events after vaccinations. In 1999, for example, the programme recorded several reports, not particularly significant on the statistical level, which suggested how in some cases the RotaShield vaccine, against the rotavirus, caused severe alterations of the digestive system: subsequent epidemiological studies proved the effective causal relationship and the vaccine was immediately withdrawn from the market. In another case, in 1998, the VAERS reported a potential slight increase in the Guillain–Barré syndrome (GBS, an autoimmune disease which affects the peripheral nerve system and respiratory muscles) in people to whom the Menactra meningococcal conjugate vaccine had been administered. In order to investigate this relationship, various studies were carried out, including two broad studies which, after having analysed a population of over two million vaccinated adolescents, proved the absence of any link between the two events (Yih et al. 2012). In actual fact, the hypothesized relationship between vaccines and GBS had already emerged in 1976–1977 when, after a campaign of anti-flu vaccination following a pandemic of swine flu (H1N1), an increase in the cases of GBS was observed in the United States. In this case too, subsequent epidemiological studies proved no correlation or a weak one, which does not exceed three cases out of a million administrations (Galeotti et al. 2013). Therefore, overall, the data that emerge from the VAERS confirm the efficacy of the widespread network of control and the very low risks of the vaccines.[5]

The second control centre is in Europe, in Geneva, at the head office of the WHO. Here, in 1999, a specific scientific committee, the *Global Advisory Committee on Vaccine Safety* (GACVS), was set up, designed to provide a series of authoritative and independent scientific advice on the safety and monitoring of vaccines, of global or regional interest, also with the purpose of making the short- and long-term national immunization programmes more effective. One of the first guarantees of independence is its composition. The GACVS has 14 members, all strictly without conflicts of interest, selected in such a way as

---

[5] VAERS, http://tinyurl.com/lbxf3k8

to guarantee a fair geographical and gender representation and above all, chosen from experts of international standing in a wide range of disciplines, such as epidemiology, statistics, paediatrics, general medicine, pharmacology and toxicology, infectious diseases, public health, immunology, vaccinology, pathology, ethics, neurology, regulation and drug safety. These members, including the president, remain in office for an initial period of 3 years, which may be renewed only once. The operating role of the committee, which meets every 3 months to report to the bodies of the WHO, consists of "providing advice on urgent questions, if necessary", including: evaluating any causal relations between the vaccines (and/or their components) and the adverse events attributed to them; creating, where necessary an ad hoc task force with the task of monitoring and evaluating adequate methodological and empirical studies on any form of presumed association between vaccines or components and adverse events; constantly monitoring the most recent and meticulous literature, from basic science to epidemiology, on the safety of the vaccines (global or regional); providing scientific recommendations aimed at helping the *Strategic Advisory Group of Experts* (SAGE) for vaccines and immunization of the WHO—in collaboration with the national governments and international organizations—to develop policies on problems of vaccine safety, with particular attention to developing countries.[6] From the documents of the meetings—of which the archive is available online, confirming the sensitivity of the board to the greatest social fears on topics such as the relationship between the trivalent MMR and autism, immunological overload and the harmfulness of adjuvants—the vaccines emerge regularly as cleared.[7] In 2011, the GACVS set up a simplified global system, also designed for the emerging countries, to collect the reports of adverse events from vaccines (AEFI, *Adverse Events Following Immunization*) which is easy to access and compile via the Internet.[8]

These monitoring systems—international, public, transparent and subject to control by citizens—offer a mass of unequivocal data, collected on tens of millions of individuals, on the tiny risks of vaccines. Beyond cognitive biases, each evaluation of risk (as argued several times) makes sense only in relation to the benefits and risks offered by alternative strategies; therefore, if compared with other drugs—for example, aspirin or antibiotics—vaccines entail definitely lower risks, arriving first absolutely on safety. Lastly, let's have a look at

---

[6] WHO. The Global Advisory Committee on Vaccine Safety, http://tinyurl.com/gl29vm8
[7] WHO. Global Vaccine Safety, List of Topics Covered in Our Committee Meetings, http://tinyurl.com/hep7hp4
[8] WHO. Global Vaccine Safety, http://tinyurl.com/hep7hp4

the relations between risks and benefits. In the case of measles, it is known that the natural virus causes the death of an individual every 2000/3000 people infected, while the vaccine may cause one encephalitis out of a million administrations—a percentage so rare on the statistical level as to place it at the limit of the effective causal relationship. While pertussis causes death in one case out of 100 of infections (one encephalitis out of 20 and one pneumonia out of 18) , the vaccine can cause from 0 to 10 encephalopathies every million administrations; tetanus causes 3 deaths out of 100 infected individuals, the vaccine at the most creates convulsions which are not severe (with recovery) in one case out of 2000; meningitis causes death in one case out of 10 (and in almost 3 out of 10 babies, where it is frequent), while the vaccine, at the most, causes a transitory insensitivity of the limbs in one case out of 10,000. Lastly, the vaccines for mumps and rubella have no risks or contraindications, while the natural forms of these diseases cause, respectively, encephalitis (at times sterility) and the death of the foetus in pregnancy (Mantovani and Florianello 2016).

It is not an advantageous ratio or an unequal fight: there is no comparison between the high risks, at times lethal, that are run by not being vaccinated and those tiny risks which there could be if vaccinated. Those who avoid vaccinations out of fear of these insignificant figures should avoid more probable risks such using a car, household cleaning products, various foods (peanuts, eggs, shellfish, etc.) and almost all drugs, should not smoke or drink alcohol and, naturally, hope not to be affected by any of the infections just mentioned.

## The Therapeutic Vaccines of the Future: Cancer and Neurodegenerative Diseases

The most important scientific revolution in the field of vaccinology in the past 20 years is owed to the Italian researcher Rino Rappuoli who has effectively founded a new disciplinary branch: *reverse vaccinology*. From the Chinese court officials, via Jenner and Pasteur, the logic of the manufacturers of vaccines has always been to find or produce an attenuated form starting from a natural pathogenic agent to then inoculate it into a healthy person in order to obtain the production of antibodies and immunity without the risks of the disease. Today, thanks to the advances made on the level of knowledge and technologies in the field of molecular biology, it is possible to design vaccines "at the drawing board", i.e. starting from computational information on the genomics and structure of the pathogenic agent, as well as of the parts that can react with the human immune system, such as to create an essential and specific (and so safer and more effective) vaccine for the molecular components of the microorganisms. After having created between 1989 and 1996 the first acellular recombinant vaccine (which unlike the previous vaccines does not contain cells but only fragments of the bacterium), against pertussis, Rappuoli—in collaboration with Craig Venter, the American biologist known for having directed one of the two centres which made possible the sequencing of the Human Genome Project—succeeded in producing in 2000 the first vaccine designed starting from the information in the genome of the microorganism: the meningococcus of serogroup B. In Europe, this holds some of the greatest responsibility for infantile deaths caused by meningitis, a very aggressive bacterium, usually resistant to treatment with antibiotics. In 1991, Rappuoli was the only European researcher to be awarded the prestigious Paul Ehrlich and Ludwig Darmstaedter Prize, the most important recognition, established in 1952, in the field of vaccinology.

Reverse vaccinology then extended its field of research, embracing structural vaccinology (based on genomic, structural and computational investigations of the microorganisms), synthetic biology (which allows designing and manufacturing existing biological components and systems or ones that do not yet exist in nature) and the molecular development of the adjuvants. These represent a field in which immunology and vaccinology have not been greatly engaged in recent decades—an oversight which is showing its limits, as shown by the recent case of the inactivated trivalent influenza vaccine (TIV). A decade ago, this vaccine risked being abandoned because, especially in children, it showed a low efficiency (equal to 43%) but the development of new and safe adjuvant molecule (MF59) was able to increase its efficiency up to 86%, proving that in some cases the role of the adjuvant is equal to that of the vaccine itself (Vesikari et al. 2011).

The inefficacy of a vaccine is often linked to its low capacity to produce immunological memory, forcing the population to have continuous and expensive booster doses and that of the immunological memory is also a topic of vaccinology of the future. Not all vaccines offer lifelong coverage. Many, as in the case of the trivalent DTP, cyclically need booster injections—a fact which, especially in emerging countries, where the availability of doses and the health organizations are deficient, significantly reduces the possibility of reaching the expected thresholds of herd immunity. The weakness of the immunological memory may, however, also be due to other factors. It may be caused, for example, by a continuous change of the appearances of surface of the viruses which, preventing the immune system from "focusing" on the enemy to defeat, causes in the immune cells the absence of memory of past encounters with the virus. The chase and reciprocal adaptation between the immune system and pathogenic agents is similar to that between predators and their prey: not only do the cells of the immune system continue to differentiate themselves (in order to recognize the highest number of potential invaders), but the surfaces of the viruses do the same, as in the typical case of HIV and seasonal viruses, to avoid being recognized. We have to be vaccinated against seasonal viruses every year because the surface proteins vary and, although belonging to the same strain, from one year to the next the human organism does not recognize them. Recently, however, structural vaccinology has identified stable parts of the seasonal influenza virus, based on the hypothesis that, due to the very fact of belonging to a given strain, each virus possesses constant and distinctive structural elements: identifying them and directing them against a vaccine would be a great success. The experimental work seems promising and the expectations are to succeed in covering the population from influenza viruses for several years with a single vaccine. This would be a great economic and health advantage for everyone, especially for children and the elderly, the two categories typically at greatest risk.

With respect to that of young or mature individuals, the immunological memory of the elderly has proven to be much weaker. This is a fact which sometimes renders the vaccinations vain (Franceschi et al. 2000). Offering vaccines with a "reinforced memory" to these subjects would protect a fragile and growing part of th Western population. In this sense, in the coming years, the mechanisms of the immunological memory and more in general the articulated relationship of interactions between the molecules of the vaccines and the variegated world of the immunomodulating cells and molecules of the immune system will be studied in further depth. For example, the interesting mechanism whereby some vaccines succeed in offering coverage not only to the microorganism to which they are directed but also, with a beneficial spillover effect, for microorganisms belonging to similar, dissimilar or completely different families still remains uncertain—this is the case, for example, of the BCG vaccine against tuberculosis, which also immunizes against leprosy—a phenomenon known as heterologous or degenerate immunity (Mason et al. 2015).

Another theoretical gap to be filled will be to understand, and exploit, the role of the line of "innate" or nonspecific immune defence, essentially based on macrophages (cells that digest extraneous organisms or damaged or waste tissue). With the exception of that for yellow fever, all the vaccines produced to date interact with the "adaptive" and nonspecific line of defence or with the cells that coadjuvate or produce the antibodies against the invaders. By doing so, however, only half the "team" available has been used, leaving on the sidelines players that are potentially of the top level that have proven that they can defend the organism from external aggressions perfectly well. The difficulty of obtaining vaccines against AIDS, hepatitis C and malaria—in this last case, in 2014 a vaccine capable of protecting 50% of children from contagion was tested and about 30% of them from severe episodes of the disease (Mantovani and Florianello 2016, p. 52)—is probably due to the little research on this neglected line of immune defence. The research group of Riccardo Cortese, the Italian researcher who has developed one of the vaccines against Ebola, now in the phase of experimentation, has started to work on this line. For example, the idea was to develop vaccines not from fragments but from the whole Ebola virus, attenuating it through the insertion in a vector virus (adenovirus): this is a strategy which allows the immune system of the host organism not only to develop antibodies with the cellular line of adaptive defence but also to aggress the virus with the cells of the innate line of defence (in particular, the lymphocytes T and NK killer cells), capable of recognizing and destroying the infectious agent missed by the antibodies.

Lastly, the scientific community agrees in seeing the future of vaccinology not only in preventive vaccines but also in therapeutic ones. It has to be said that these are stationary at an elementary phase of experimentation. The two lines of research taken so far concern therapeutic oncological vaccines, capable of activating the human immune system towards some parts of the tumour or to regulate the inflammatory activity of the carcinogenic context, and therapeutic vaccines for generative diseases such as arteriosclerosis, Alzheimer's disease, Huntington's Chorea and Parkinson's disease, in which the vaccines could direct the immune system towards the molecules that foster the degeneration of the brain tissues (Luthi-Carter 2003; Yong et al. 2011; Evans et al. 2014; Ramsingh et al. 2015).

In the first two decades of the twentieth century, the enthusiasm and funds for research on vaccines gave a marvellous boost to research, which in about 30 years produced 20 or so vaccines capable of fighting the most important infectious diseases in the history of humanity. Society has changed and, as the concept of pathocenosis suggests, we are now oriented towards a new ratio of balance with the environment and so with new chronic diseases emerging due to well-being. In the next 20 years, we could replicate the successes of the past, but although having a potentially effective instrument like reverse vaccinology in our hands, the society of the future might not use it, precisely due to well-being which not infrequently rekindles irrationality, attenuating the principle of reality and the desire for knowledge.

# 6

## Conclusions

## A New Alliance Between Scientists and Citizens for a Knowledge Society

In the United States, according to a study by the University of Stanford, 82% of North American high school students are incapable of correctly evaluating the credibility of the information found on the Internet, i.e. they are unable to distinguish the authenticity of an image or understand whether a text is sponsored and base their trust not on the origin and authority of the sources but on how much the news is shared and on the "likes" it receives. This is a result which the authors themselves define "dismaying", "bleak" and "[a] threat to democracy" (Stanford 2016).[1] In Europe, a recent French survey reports that 51% of French citizens are interested in conspiracy topics, and 36% of young people between the ages of 15 and 24 believe that there really exists an occult society which governs the world, a figure which pushed the government, represented by the former French Minister of Education Najat Vallaud-Belkacem, to inaugurate in 2016 a campaign for schools entitled "You're being manipulated!" (*On te manipule!*), conceived to raise the awareness of pupils and teachers in schools, with ad hoc educational material (media literacy).[2] Western society and the most advanced democracies have to face a great challenge over the next three decades, which is to find a way to handle the

---

[1] Stanford History Education Group, (Nov 22, 2016) Evaluation Information: The Cornerstone of Civic Online Reasoning. https://sheg.stanford.edu/upload/V3LessonPlans/Executive%20Summary%2011.21.16.pdf

[2] https://www.gouvernement.fr/on-te-manipule

© Springer International Publishing AG, part of Springer Nature 2018
A. Grignolio, *Vaccines: Are they Worth a Shot?*, https://doi.org/10.1007/978-3-319-68106-1_6

**137**

information overload, learning to manage the perception of risk and manipulated news.

This is a challenge to which the very ability for survival of these societies is linked. Various indicators suggest that in 2050 the world will probably have to feed more than nine billion people, that in Europe and the United States the number of individuals suffering from neurodegenerative diseases and senile dementia will triple and that population density, especially in the metropolises, will double. This means more food, less waste of water and energy and more effective medicine, prevention and drugs. The only way to achieve these objectives is to rely on scientific and technological development, but we cannot leave scientists alone in the face of enormous responsibilities like this, nor continue dialoguing with them as we have done so far, that is by raising irrational doubts and underpaying (especially in Italy) their research. The scientific community is unanimous in maintaining that increased food production will come about only thanks to the development of biotechnologies applied to agriculture, i.e. GMOs, the only ones today already able to increase the yield per hectare, saving water, solar energy, cultivable land, fertilizers, pesticides and to better resist in contexts of drought or flooding. Scientists agree in saying that the emissions of greenhouse gas and pollutants have to be reduced, to focus instead on a production of energy with a low environmental impact. Lastly, all the researchers in the biomedical field maintain that to obtain increasingly effective and personalized drugs, animal experimentation still has to be used, concentrating on the genomic analysis of the population and developing new preventive and therapeutic vaccines, capable of facing up to the effects of enormous migratory flows and high inhabitant concentrations. Apart from a general consensus for renewable energies, on all the other issues—GMOs, animal experimentation, disclosure of genomic data and vaccines—a growing part of Western society expresses perplexity or even actual opposition, and opposition, as mentioned in the first chapter, comes precisely from the most educated and affluent part of society, therefore from the potentially most influential part from a political and economic point of view. Never as today, should we accept the challenges of progress in a rational, disenchanted and authentic way, tackling open-faced even the risks on the path of innovation. We, therefore, have to review the relations between scientists and citizens to reduce these misunderstandings, in the name of a future alliance based on dialogue and comprehension. How? By meeting halfway between science and society and with a solution that takes account of recent history and of the solutions offered by scientific research.

Recent history suggests in the first place that scientists have not always been able to correctly communicate their ideas and needs to society. Apart from notable and important exceptions, the scientific community is too often shut up in its laboratories, heedless of the fundamental importance of being able to communicate the values of science. This task has gradually been left to a separate community, that of those who raise popular awareness of science, who have not always been able to interpret these values. For decades, raising popular awareness of science was the prerogative of professional figures trained in the so-called Departments of Science, Technology and Society (STS), focused on a sociological approach characterized by an anti-scientist attitude. Their philosophical mentality rested on a—radically sceptical—postmodern, relativist and narrative vision of science, in which science is seen as one of many social practices, capable of producing stories, myths, narrations or descriptions of reality which are neither more authentic nor more reliable and objective than other human activities. In essence, science was seen as one "opinion" amongst the many available and facts, data, evidence and objectivity were ignored or ridiculed because they were considered a fictitious phenomenon (including in the sense of fiction "story of fiction"), one of the many consequences of social, cultural and economic constructs of our time. In such a perspective, scientists are considered individuals guided exclusively by biased interests, influenced by the "powers that be" and "big industry". This approach to science has favoured in society the assertion of the opinion that a principle of objectivity and demonstrability in reality does not exist that allows distinguishing between true, false and fictive, and one of its consequences is that today on the Internet the theories proved by data and experts and any interpretation or belief whatsoever are equivalent, since everyone, according to the relativist approach, has the right to claim their own convictions. As the historian Carlo Ginzburg was the first to demonstrate in a masterly way, the dissolution of the concept of "proof" is owed to the recovery of Nietzsche by a certain culture of the left in the 1970s. The Nietzschean idea that objectivity was illusory and truth, a mobile army of metaphors was multiplied by the post-modernists, who made it the banner of their relativist theories naively aimed at tolerance. The beliefs of subordinate, ex-colonial and tribal cultures, like scientific theories, were considered equivalent interpretations of reality. They were years when the authority of competences was taken for authoritarianism and terms such as reality, objectivity and fact were considered dynamics of power of reactionary thought. It has taken more than 30 years to understand that it was a great misunderstanding. The crazy theories of the negationists à la Faurisson who deny the existence of the Nazis' gas chambers use the same instruments that once were those of relativists and constructivists of a progressive character (Ginzburg 2000, 2006). When there is no objective reality, or a method to distinguish if what is stated corresponds to it or not—but all the narrations of reality are valid, independently of the correspondence of facts and evidence—then it becomes possible to believe in the reality of conspiracies, of the negationist or of the charlatan, just as scientific reality based on evidence is believed.

The academic and cultural success of postmodern relativism, which until a few years ago inspired science popularization, has certainly not helped the new generations understand, for example, whether GMOs do good or bad, whether vaccines create autism or not or whether animal experimentation is still necessary. These three issues, we have seen, are essential for the social development of the coming decades, and maintained by the greatest world experts in the sector, as well as data and evidence of the most accredited international literature. Yet the sites that deform, falsify and invent data and images to negate their benefits are equal or greater than the authentic ones. If in reality we have different ways, including perceptive, to distinguish and find our way around the true-false-fictive trio, in the Internet everything becomes more difficult, and the competences required are greater—and the gap between scientists and citizens risks becoming even wider.

Today, fortunately, things are changing. The fashion of STS has worn off and has given way to solid schools of scientific popularization where scientists and humanists discuss facts, scientific discoveries and ethical values at stake, without (or almost) ideologies and preconceptions, but it will still take time before these new generations of popularizers succeed in delivering a different social perception of science—before a generalized mistrust of scientists ends and the idea that science and democracy share multiple methodological and ethical-political aims (Corbellini 2011). The refusal of authority, the respect of the facts, the transparency of criticism, the freedom of communication and access to results are some values fought for by science and then assimilated by democracy. They are in the articles of association of the first scientific societies established at the dawn of the scientific revolution which, during the Enlightenment, allowed countries such as England, the United States, the Netherlands, Germany, Italy and France (in the last three in a more fluctuating way) to develop generalized knowledge and well-being never achieved before in the history of humanity. The scientific revolution acted as an impulse for the democratic revolution and various minds were strongly influenced by this knowledge—Franklin, Jefferson, Montesquieu, as well as several members of the British House of Lords—involved directly in the revolutions which led to the formulation of fundamental human rights. Later, between the eighteenth and nineteenth centuries, the countries that believed in the progress offered by the scientific method reached the best socio-economic parameters—i.e. the number of murders and the rate of corruption decreased, and per capita wealth, the average life expectancy of citizens and freedom of the press increased. It is an exciting path, recently confirmed by Asian countries like Taiwan, South Korea and Singapore, which have focused on science, technology and innovation, at the same time increasing many of their socio-cultural and hygiene-health parameters. In other words, investing in science is the surest way of ensuring an improvement in the indexes linked to employment, well-being, longevity and good practices of social co-existence. This message—or rather this fact supported by evidence—paradoxically has not yet been passed on to the general public and politics: a shortcoming for which the popularizers above all are responsible. A great deal of work still remains to be done, especially in Italy.

On the common path that leads to a new alliance between science and society, alongside the steps that the popularizers must take, there are naturally those that the scientists must take. Until a few years ago, the greatest criticism of them, not without reason, was that of staying in their ivory towers, of using excessively specialized language and offering only "cold data"; in other words, they were accused of being without that irony, emotion and warmth which today we know is necessary for the successful narration of a scientific adventure. The Observa 2014 data, as mentioned at the beginning, indicate an inversion of the trend, seeing that they observe both an improvement in the perception of science by Italian citizens and a greater participation by scientists—with the public recognizing their growing credibility—in the increasingly numerous festivals of science. As well as coming out of their laboratories more often to meet the general public, they should also be more conscious of and responsible for the cognitive imbalance due to the competences.

The fragmentation of scientific disciplines has created a highly specialized network of competences which find it hard to dialogue with one another and with the different social players: in a democracy, this creates an asymmetrical relationship of power by virtue of which those who know end up by imposing their decisions while citizens, and often the politicians, can only trust them. Researchers in the biomedical field are, therefore, asked to make more effort, as they deal with treatment, diseases, the body of the patient and, lastly, with pain. If it is not acceptable that the patients impose on the doctor their therapeutic course, it is equally inadmissible that the doctor abuses the exclusivity of their scientific knowledge. Similar, age-old relations of strength are no longer valid today, as the actors at play have changed since mass education and the Internet have made patients potentially capable of taking part in some of the decisions in the therapeutic field.

The effort towards open discussion, based on data and comprehensible evidence, must be made by scientists to politics as well. Abroad, in recent years, in this field specific professional figures have emerged, known as *science advisors*: these are scientists who, without conflicts of interest decide to put themselves at the service of the institutions, acting as intermediaries between the scientific community and political decisions, offering consulting services, suggesting fields of development for innovation and stemming the numerous pseudoscientific proposals and frauds to which the state bodies (not last the Italian Parliament) are often subject. The Presidency of the European Commission had this figure (Chief Scientific Advisor) until 2014; various Presidents of the United States, up to Barack Obama, regularly used a *science advisor* (who can also count on a group of advisors on topics of science and technology, the PCAST); in the United Kingdom, every government department has a scientific advisor, coordinated by an office (the Government Office for Science) which informs the Prime Minister, and Australia and New Zealand have also developed various political offices for *science advisors*. This healthy proximity between the worlds of science and politics in the English-speaking world has allowed the development of a new stimulating theoretical approach, *evidence-based policy*, which uses the methodology coming from clinical trials to evaluate the government's actions, using statistics, establishing clear objectives evaluated by independent committees, imposing controls in the different phases of development, refinancing only effective projects and adopting a public and transparent system for costs and communication (Young et al. 2002; Rosenstock and Lee 2002; Majcen 2016). If many other countries were to acquire similar instruments, they could gain greatly from them.

Lastly, after the popularizers, scientists and politicians, there remain the citizens: it is they, all of us, who are asked to make the most significant step. As anticipated in the first chapter, the citizens will be increasingly exposed to an information load on crucial questions relative to health, work economic and political decisions; these are delicate issues in which they will be informed by the media and the Internet, where there is an indistinct ocean of real, fake, manipulated and contradictory and above all potentially dangerous information. If, in the coming decades, we do not acquire the cognitive instruments to find our way around a similar maze of information, we will endanger the development of society and the very continuation of our democracy: it will be a difficult challenge, during which we will have to show that we can overcome once again, the limits imposed by our evolutionary past. If, on the one hand, citizens today can access all the information possible concerning their choices; on the other they have a neurocognitive structure which has inherited the limits imposed by a very different evolutionary past: the evolutionists define the context we are in as *misfit, mismatched* or *maladapted* to modernity. Managing the complexity of current information with a brain that developed in the savannah of the Pleistocene is like mounting modern software (for example Windows 7) on old hardware (e.g. the Commodore 64) of the early 1980s: the risk that the computer "crashes" is fairly high. We have to give our cerebral machine new instruments to make it capable of managing the more complex programs imposed by today's society of knowledge. Let's have a brief look at the conceptual instruments necessary for the society of coming years and the suggestions that emerge to face, in particular, the rejection of vaccination.

In the first place, we have to deal with the consequences of bounded rationality. The prospect theory worked out by Daniel Kahneman and Amos Tversky, we have seen, suggests that the decisions of citizens tend to be irrational and suboptimal. In particular, when we have to choose between different alternatives, we have such an aversion to risk that we end up by evaluating it erroneously, focusing on marginal and improbable events or confusing the context and variables at stake. That is not all. Kahneman has also shown the presence of two different thought processes: one fast, intuitive and emotive one (system 1) which often leads us towards the wrong choices, and a slower, but logical and reflective one (system 2) which tends to suggest more correct evaluations (Tversky and Kahneman 1974; Kahneman and Tversky 1996; Kahneman 2012). Subsequently, this theory was supplemented by the research of another important psychologist, Gerd Gigerenzer, who balanced the evaluative errors of the two systems by observing how the capacity to choose of the reflective system is compromised by its limited capacity to memorize data, and the intuitive system in many contexts is more efficient than thought, especially of the individuals are offered notions of statistics. Gigerenzer has also proven that in daily choices, especially in the health and financial contexts, citizens confuse the concept of risk and that of uncertainty, with often dramatic outcomes—as shown by the mistaken economic evaluations on the recent market crisis and the inability to evaluate the rate of survival in oncological diagnoses (Gigerenzer 1996, 2009, 2015; Gigerenzer and Gray 2013).

Both authors, therefore, maintain that in today's society, individuals take decisions in contexts dominated by risk and uncertainty, appealing to a limited cognitive apparatus (information, time, memory, etc.), which makes them decide using a limited number of mental shortcuts (heuristic approach) instead of sophisticated rational processes. Neuroscience and evolutionary psychology today confirm that *Homo sapiens* cannot be totally rational because during evolution his bran was selected to develop intuitive behaviour and reasoning that were useful in the context of hostile life which lasted for thousands of years. These adaptations, useful in the past, are today the cause of systematic distortions of judgement (bias): the evolutionary environmental pressures have selected our brain to flee from predators, cooperate for hunting and the care of children, interact with small and hierarchical groups of individuals (tribal structure), compete with rival bands and take short-term decisions based on data that is not very complex. Today, the same brain is wired to a body which no longer has problems of survival or food, lives in metropolises which are not divided into castes, takes long or very long-term complicated decisions and has to handle an immense overload of information which also includes risky, contradictory and manipulated information. It is by comparing this huge amount of information with the two mental systems, intuitive and rational, that over the years the biases that are produced by our recurring perceptive distortions have emerged. The best known—and useful for understanding the refusal of vaccination (some already discussed in the text)—are confirmation bias, i.e. the tendency to seek confirmation of one's beliefs and refuse the contrasting evidence (according to the principle of falsification typical of the scientific method; the backfire effect, which explains why those who have very entrenched ideas on a given topic, if put in front of evidence and data which prove its falsity, instead of changing their minds reinforce their erroneous convictions; the group bias, which is the tendency to favour the people belonging to the social group in which one lives and sharing the ideas in it (in agreement with the notion of cultural cognition of Dan Kahan); the omission bias, which proves how in contexts of a risky choice, i.e. when you are in front of an alternative between a concrete action and an omission, there is a tendency to choose the omission even when it exposes to greater risks, or the tendency to judge the consequences of the natural course of events (severe effects of the infectious disease) as more acceptable compared to the consequences of a human intervention (negligible adverse reactions, when present, of the vaccination); the finalistic bias which consists of attributing a purpose to behaviour or facts guided by chance; the neglect of probability bias, i.e. the inability to understand real dangers and risks that make us over-evaluate the innocuous ones and underestimate the more dangerous ones; the bias of illusory correlations, which is the tendency to confuse correlation and causation, and which makes us associate two events which are distinct; and lastly, the memory or response bias—greatly studied as a systematic error in epidemiology—which shows how in questionnaires for clinical records patients or their relatives remember incorrectly the behaviour that preceded the onset of a disease according to the (aetiological) causes deemed responsible.

In the second place, this type of knowledge would have to be delivered to the field of actions of the government: the new acquisitions in cognitive psychology and neuroscience make us more lucid but also, potentially, more fragile. If used responsibly, bounded rationality, cognitive biases and emotional thought can become a powerful instrument to guide citizens towards choices that are correct, useful and effective for society; but if they are used in a manipulating way they can become a pure instrument of coercion for commercial, demagogical, populist or propaganda purposes. The citizens of the knowledge society, also thanks to the use of the Internet, are being oriented towards increasingly direct forms of democracy, such as deliberative or participatory. In this context, they will be constantly involved in complex decision-making processes on crucial questions linked to work, health insurance, medical therapies and financial strategies (Beccaria and Grignolio 2014). Some countries are already getting ready, with the United Kingdom in first place: for its campaign of reforms, the Cameron government drew inspiration from a book on cognitive neuroscience, *Nudge: Improving Decisions about Health, Wealth, and Happiness* (Thaler and Sunstein 2008), to exploit the knowledge of cognitive-behavioural factors which influence the decisions of citizens to promote virtuous and socially useful conduct. Thaler received the Nobel Prize for Economics in 2017, confirming the growing interest of science in behavioural economics and cognitive neuroscience, which study the architecture of social decisions. This Prize followed those awarded in 2002 to Khaneman and in 1978 to Herbert A. Simon, the father of bounded rationality. Included in the structure of the British government in 2010, the *nudge unit*, then part of the Behavioural Insights Team, has performed in these years work aimed at decreasing expenses and making bureaucracy more efficient, sending personalized letters to tax evaders, reminding citizens late in their tax payments with messages that exploited social reciprocity, increasing the participation in institutional initiatives by attaching the invitation to a lottery with small prizes to be won, and eliminating the errors of medical prescriptions thanks to simplified and precompiled forms. In 2015, the President of the United States, Obama, also established a "nudge unit" at the White House and so did the Australian government recently. The idea of the "nudge" comes from the fact that, in the architecture of the choices of individuals, instead of prohibiting or imposing choices to improve people's well-being, the institutions can also obtain appreciable results merely by orienting the choices in the right direction: instead of banning junk food, the "nudge theory" maintains, it is sufficient to put healthy food within smelling distance and in the right places. It is about keeping the freedom of choice of the citizens, replacing orders by cognitively oriented incentives. Thaler and Sunstein define this approach *libertarian paternalism*. They are all instruments capable of offering citizens an active role in the phases of political discussion—and the same applies for the choices that concern science and innovation, always on condition (and this is essential) that there is an assumption of responsibility and the scientific method is adopted. Anyone who wants to take part in the debate may do so, but based not on mere "hearsay" but on the method and knowledge of the facts, on pain of exclusion. Acquiring knowledge and method will also be of use to citizens to avoid potential abuse of these instruments, and this opens up to the last point of the new alliance between science and society.

Thirdly, it will be opportune to start teaching the new generations our cognitive limits and the instruments to supersede them, including them in educational syllabi. This is what James Flynn, the most authoritative living psychologist of intelligence, advises: after having proven that the intelligence quotient increased during the twentieth century (the so-called Flynn effect) thanks to the free and stimulating environments created by science and technology in the Western democracies, in his recent research he has analysed the minimum instruments of thought to give to a youngster so that they can understand critically, and appreciate, modernity—a modernity that is made increasingly incomprehensible both by a growing abstraction of disciplinary knowledge and different anti-modernity and anti-scientist demands and ideologies. Flynn, in essence, has analysed which are the most frequent biases that prevent us from understanding today's reality and which are the most rational and critical cognitive instruments through which future citizens can overcome them and be able to make more effective and morally better choices in the interest of people and society (Flynn has always declared he is a progressive thinker). To obtain a similar result, he believes it is necessary to teach 20 "key concepts" in schools and universities, including: how the economic market works, how a statistical sample is constructed, what the difference is between correlation and causation, what the placebo effect is, what the criterion of falsifiability, a control group, a percentage and a proportion are, how the intelligence quotient (IQ) is measured and lastly, how to avoid the cognitive errors and logical fallacies represented by relativism, anti-realism, finalism and explanations that instrumentally use recourse to nature for justification (naturist fallacy). It will have been noticed that many of these instruments would be useful to demolish several of the criticisms of vaccines. For Flynn, the social environment has to be sufficiently varied and free to allow the genetic predispositions, more or less promising in each individual, to be able to be fulfilled in a fair way, and he reaches the conclusion that although "thinking critically has never represented an automatic guarantee of power, anyone who has the 20 key concepts will be able to count on a liberated mind without which no personal autonomy is possible" (Flynn 2013).

## Some Instruments for an Effective Communication Strategy on Anti-vaccination Resistance

Let us now look at how all these studies have been used to explain the social resistance against vaccines—and have offered the instruments to overcome them, with at times highly effective results, starting from a brief summary of the conclusions reached by neuroscience, cognitive and evolutionary psychology, epidemiological and demographic analyses and the strategies of health communication on the reasons that today fuel the false beliefs and the possible risks.

In the first place, it has been understood that, counter-intuitively, it is above all the most educated and affluent part of the population that rejects vaccinations. The reasons, as amply underlined, are due to the fact that it is that group which is most informed about the possible adverse reactions; it often uses the Internet and the social networks as an instrument of in-depth study and, therefore, is exposed to an overload of information based on false and contradictory notions and linked to the risk. This is a context which in the decision-making process and in the evaluation of the health choices induces refusing the risk, the mistaken overestimation of which is based on statistically insignificant data—while the information relative to the low risks and benefits are underestimated. In addition, this section of the population is often oriented, by cultural and economic status, towards a sound healthy-living approach which today is dominated by a fallacious naturist ideology (in general characterized by organic diets and the use of homeopathic treatments or "alternative" medicines) which looks at vaccinations with suspicion or aversion. This way, a system of beliefs is formed which is constantly reinforced by cognitive mechanisms. In turn, these regulate the sharing of these political–cultural values which obey tribal dynamics and the idea of belonging (or desiring or believing to belong) to an elite social group. In addition, there is the growing rate of low and late fertility which characterizes the most advanced societies of the Western world. Advanced age parents are effectively more exposed to the risk of diseases of the baby, the uncertainty of the outcome of the birth and the danger of not having other chances of reproduction, and live for the first years of care of their offspring in a psychic, professional and existential phase, tending to be stressful and dissatisfying. This creates an overall context which fosters the perceptive distortions in the evaluation of the risks on the health and medical choices to which to submit their children and which induces parents to reduce or avoid anxiety-inducing situations in communications with healthcare operators. In addition to these reasons, there are radical social changes, such as the spread of disinformation via the Internet and a weakening of the authority of the figure of the doctor due to a misunderstood interpretation of the autonomy of the patient. The studies that have taken into account this new scientific and cultural evidence have carried out interesting experiments which offer useful ideas on how to better structure public communication in order to intercept and orient the undecided and even the radical opponents towards rational decision regarding vaccines.

Given that the prospect theory shows the human tendency to accept the risk in a context of possible losses, in contrast with the aversion to risk in a context of possible gain, and given that for a part of the population vaccines are perceived as risky, vaccination should be promoted explaining what could be lost if this risk were not taken, instead of explaining what we could gain. In other words, in communication on vaccines, it is much more important to emphasize the protection lost in relation to potentially fatal diseases in the case of refusal, delivering messages and stories that explain the high risks, rather than insisting on their efficacy and safety. Hesitant parents, therefore, have to be reminded that vaccinating their child with, let's say, the trivalent MMR will protect it from these three specific diseases, giving lifelong protection which will make the parents less anxious and more confident (Abhyankar et al. 2008; Ball et al. 1998).

Appealing to the general social benefits connected with vaccination also seems to be particularly ineffective, for example the importance of herd immunity: the most effective instrument proved to be the communication to parents of the risks of disease and the advantages of vaccination referred to their specific child, focusing on safety and family values, and on the instinct of protecting one's children. Communications should, therefore, be as personalized and nominal as possible, as far as the risks/benefits of the individual children and the effects of the individual diseases are concerned (Hendrix et al. 2014).

Lastly, two recent important experiments have been conducted which suggest further key elements of an effective communication on vaccination especially with that fringe of parents who radically refuse it. The first experiment, aimed at evaluating the efficacy of the messages to reduce wrong perceptions and increase the diffusion of the trivalent MMR vaccine, was published in 2014 in the well-known journal "Pediatrics". 1759 U.S. parents and adults with children under the age of 17 were interviewed and subjected to four different types of information: one focused on the absence of evidence of the relationship between trivalent and autism; one that made use of texts in which the risks of three diseases preventable with the trivalent were explained; one that used images of children suffering from the three diseases and one which used a dramatic story written by a mother about her son who is dying from measles. This information should have been effective, contemplating some communication strategies suggested by the neuroscientific and psychological knowledge discussed here: emphasis on the risks of the loss of health and the use of personalized and emotionally engaging stories and images. Yet none of this information had a positive influence on the decision to vaccinate their children or not. Surprisingly, the authors underlined that although the communication delivered in the experiment had succeeded in convincing some parents of the fact that the trivalent does not cause autism, it did not reduce their opposition to the vaccines. In addition, the most adverse fringe, after the experiment, even showed a greater refusal. The authors concluded maintaining that the attempts to "correct false and wrong ideas about vaccines can be particularly counterproductive" (Nyhan et al. 2014).

What eluded the authors of the study was the strength of the confirmation bias and the backfire effect or that inefficacy of corrective information which is (above all) capable of making parents impermeable to any reasoning and to annul even the best practices of communication.

Starting from these presuppositions, in 2015, another experiment was carried out, this time published in "PNAS", one of the most authoritative journals in the world, in which the authors submitted a set of information to a sample of 811 individuals. On the first day, they were given a test in which they had to expose their attitude towards vaccines on a scale from 1 (very favourable) to 6 (very contrary) to then go on and express their opinion of how much they agreed in believing that vaccines caused autism. Distraction questions were then asked to avoid the participants understanding the purpose of the experiment, on some beliefs linked to euthanasia and abortion, and to make sure that they answered correctly and not approximately; only those who passed the test were called back the next day. On the second day, the participants were divided at random into three different groups. One group was asked to read the information on the risks of measles, mumps and rubella, communicated in three different ways: the story of a mother on the experience of having her child of ten months affected by an almost fatal form of measles; three photos of three children suffering from severe forms of measles, mumps and rubella; three simple warnings on how important it is to vaccinate children. Another group, on the other hand, was read a set of information aimed at *correcting* the idea that the vaccine causes autism, also showing some extracts, comprehensible and convincing, of three different scientific studies which proved the absence of any relationship. A third control group was shown cartoons. Lastly, the participants were asked to again state their attitude towards vaccination, followed by another distraction test. Finally, they were all invited to answer some questions to evaluate their past attitude to vaccinations and their future intentions on the possibility of vaccinating their children.

The experiment revealed that the group that received the corrective information on the relationship between vaccines and autism had not changed their attitude, confirming the experiment of "Pediatrics". The authors of this experiment, however, discussed in detail the reasons (eluded in the previous one) focusing their attention on the effects of the confirmation bias and backfire, capable of inducing a cognitive closure and reinforcing the initial ideas of the anti-vaccination participants. The interesting fact is that all the other participants—including the radical anti-vaccinationists—who were not contradicted or challenged in their initial beliefs, but only informed on the risks for them and their children, significantly improved their initial attitudes towards vaccinations. The authors, in essence, did not try to attack the wrong beliefs, but decided to replace the (false) fears towards vaccines with other (real) ones towards the diseases, which entail greater risks (Horne et al. 2015). A similar approach also confirms Kahneman's theory according to which human beings, precisely due to their aversion for risk, tend to accept risks only when faced with possible losses. It is, therefore, opportune to communicate to parents not so much the efficacy and safety of vaccines—if there is no perception of the infectious risk, the gains in terms of health are ignored—but to insist on the real risks of the loss of health when deprived of vaccinal protection. These strategies, which above all show objective data, as the risks of the infectious diseases are very high and at times fatal with respect to the rare and negligible adverse reactions of the vaccines, should be taken into consideration by the institutions for the promotion of public health.

To find one's way around the best communication strategies, it is opportune to look at those contexts which are not focused on the obligation of vaccination but on those oriented towards recommendation, some of which have shown that they reach a high vaccination coverage. In addition to this strategy, there are at least three other useful suggestions to efficiently manage the requests of parents who are contrary to vaccination. These are suggestions which emerge by analysing the results offered by the "nudge theory", from the example of the health policies in Australia and some North American states, as well as the solution of the British government of the late nineteenth century which emerged from the history of the anti-vaccine movements.

In advanced democracies, it is possible to give citizens a degree of freedom such as to allow them even not to vaccinate their children. However, as in every healthy democracy, a duty corresponds to every right and a responsibility to every freedom. For the parents who are contrary, various states propose some sophisticated forms of "informed dissuasion." In several cases, this takes the form of an articulated bureaucratic procedure—which would have, inter alia, the function of selecting radical convictions from the superficial and fleeting ones, according to the golden rule of the vaccinal recommendation: make vaccinal accesses easy (opt in) and refusal difficult (opt out)—in which parents are invited to read the data, the stories and look at the images relative to the real risks of the infectious diseases preventable by the vaccine and declare in writing that they had read and understood the studies and, therefore, they assume in complete awareness responsibility for submitting their child to these risks. In some cases, the informed dissenting parents have to declare that they are not opposed to their child being called by the health service to be informed, once they are adults, of the risks of not having been vaccinated—if opportunely informed, the adolescents, either because they are less influenced by the prejudices or by opposition to their parents, often decide to abide by the vaccinal calendar. A second suggestion concerns social responsibility and consists of asking anti-vaccination parents to sign the commitment in the periods of seasonal epidemics to withdraw their children from school to avoid dangerous contagions with their classmates, especially those who are immunocompromised. Lastly, as for example, is the case in Italy in the republic of San Marino, the anti-vaccination parents must take out at their own expense an insurance policy that can compensate the health costs for possible damage from contagion, thus avoiding that it is the taxpayers—who are vaccinated— who pay for the costly hospitalization of a patient who, by personal choice, has exposed himself to a risk of infection that could have been avoided with a few euros thanks to the vaccinal prophylaxis.

Alongside these restrictions, it is equally useful to consider economic incentives, as Australia is doing with the *No Jab No Pay* programme which offers only parents who abide by the vaccinal calendar tax relief or health subsidies. All the procedures discussed so far have the aim above all of increasing Confidence in vaccinations, but they would be totally insufficient if they were not accompanied by Convenience and Complacency which only efficient vaccination services for the citizen can offer, as suggested by the English-speaking model of the 3 Cs.

Beyond the correct vaccination communication strategies, the growing social resistance to vaccinations perhaps suggests something that goes beyond the question linked to vaccines. The expected dialogue between active citizenship and institutions, contemplated by the mechanisms of participatory democracy characteristic of the knowledge society, will remain a populist mirage unless we are able to educate the new generations and the political class to take decisions distinguishing between ascertained facts, irrational choices and counter-information spread by the Internet.

This incapacity in distinguishing true from fictive perhaps concerns with greater frequency the new generations, but it is certainly also a phenomenon which, as mentioned, pervades the whole of postmodern society (Ginzburg 2006). In a period like the present where the communication media produce a plethora of omnipervasive and spectacularized information (Debord 1967), it is by no means easy to discern reliable information. With respect to the previous generations, more used to sources and paper support, for the digital native generations (millennials), today's continuous decantation between true, false, fictive, typical of the digital tests on the Internet, is more difficult to discern.

The question of so-called fake news, that the diffusion by the Internet is relaunching out of all proportion, has become central in the daily debate and has driven several authoritative international papers to wonder whether it may have played a role in the most significant recent political events such as Brexit or the election of the U.S. President Donald Trump (Cillizza 2016; Freedland 2016; Drezner 2016), to wonder, in particular whether "fake news on the money spent by Great Britain for Europe (verifiable data) [can have shifted] in part the vote on its membership of the EU; or whether doubting the place of birth of an American citizen (verifiable data) [can] influence the election of the President of the United States".[3] Issues of international politics are not exempt from conspiracy fake news either if we look at the reciprocal paranoid threats between the USA, Russia and Turkey which accuse each other of conspiring to fuel international terrorism of a religious nature or influencing political victories unfavourable for adversaries.

It is no coincidence that the Oxford Dictionary decided that the key word of 2016 was *post-truth*, which defines how "circumstances in which objective facts are less influential, in the formation of public opinion, than an appeal to the emotions and personal convictions". As is known, from the Donation of Constantine to the Protocols of the Elders of Zion, fake news and propaganda have often been used to manipulate social perception and orient political choices. Post-truth, however, is something different. It is not only a communication context where emotiveness and personal convictions have the better of verifiable data, but it is a new social condition where information, although succeeding in reaching individuals, is now globalized, characterized by a never before seen speed of propagation which distributes it in viral waves and between groups of membership opposed to one another (tribal clusters) which relaunch continuous counter-information and denials which are reciprocally ignored (confirmation bias and backfire effect) where the sources are often without geography and author (and, therefore, difficult to prosecute legally) and the competences are ignored or even mocked (disintermediation and bias of the false balance) (Grignolio 2017).

Alongside the political decisions, the other significant field where post-truth is exercised is the scientific milieu (Williamson 2016; Kuntz 2017). Vaccines, GMOs, use of stem cells, animal experimentation, climate change, renewable energies and so-called alternative therapies for oncological and

---

[3] Accademia Crusca (2016), *Cos'è la post-verità?*, 19 June 2017: https://goo.gl/NdrnPf

neurodegenerative diseases are some of the topics on which in recent years the complex mechanisms of post-factual truth have appeared. These mechanisms have polluted the public debate with the diffusion of falsities and perceptions of risk which have delayed and still delay the full scientific, economic and democratic development of many advanced nations (Corbellini 2011, 2013). Of this new form of anti-intellectualism, often supported by populist deviation, we will be able to assess the outcomes only in the years to come.

Instead of stemming erroneous popular beliefs and institutional frauds, the advanced democracies ought to look to the implementation of technological innovations, the development of skills and the relaunch of scientific competition in an international context, not forgetting the epochal challenges that await us in the coming three decades. Recent political leaders and movements, both in Italy and abroad, on the other hand, form, not infrequently, their culture on the conspiracy websites, echoed by the current young generations who surf the Internet immersed in an ocean of data where real information is confused with fictitious information.

The task of citizens, schools, scientific popularization and good politics will be to react to this fatal current and develop shared strategies to distinguish democracy from the demagogical theories of conspiracy, the facts from opinions, life from fiction and truth from post-truth.

# Postface

## The Magic Thought of the Anti-vaccinationists

Vaccines are a gift to humanity of magic thought, which for some time, however, has no longer been able to recognize its paternity, that is, since science explained nature and the action of the active immunity prophylaxis. It is indeed a magic thought, as Andrea Grignolio illustrates in this book, that fuels today the false beliefs on the risks due to vaccinations.

The idea that it was possible to actively immunize an individual against a contagious disease by putting them in contact with matter produced by that disease must have circulated even before the tenth century, when in China the practice of having powder from the crusts of smallpox inhaled through the nostrils was described. Moreover, mithridatism, practised by Mithridates VI, King of Pontus in the first century AD, which consisted of acquiring immunity against some poisons, was known, and in the first century of the Vulgar Era, in the poem *Pharsalia*, Annaeus Lucanus used the term *immunitas* for the first time to describe the resistance acquired by some North African populations against the poison of snakes.

That a minimum amount of poisonous substance could be used to prevent fatal poisoning must have been even older knowledge: the nineteenth century anthropologists described various groups of nomads and breeders who in Africa practised empirical forms of active immunization of their herds, for example, wounding the animals and inserting mud mixed with a minimum quantity of fatally poisonous matter, if inoculated naturally through a bite. This is a practice which probably combines casual observations and typical elements of magic thought, in particular the laws of *sympathy* and *similarity*, as the anthropologist Marcel Mauss defined them. For the law of sympathy, the part of a thing contains all of it, especially the essence, which can, therefore, be transmitted by contagion; for the law of similarity, like acts on like, but above all cures it (*similia similibus curantur*) and at the same time chases it away, producing the opposite (law of opposition). Even though such ideas on magic are wrong, they are theories on the functioning of nature thanks to which our ancestors were able in some way to govern everyday situations, and that the observations and experiments confuted in the end, giving us a scientific explanation of the facts for which magical forces were summoned.

That there is a relationship between magic thought and immunization is shown by the attitude of some homeopaths more than a century ago. In the last two decades of the nineteenth century, while Louis Pasteur was obtaining the first immunizations with artificially attenuated infectious agents against chicken cholera, anthrax in animals and rabies in man, the clashes for and against anti-smallpox vaccination flared up again. British homeopaths were also uncertain about the question. The influential James Compton Burnett published a book entitled *Vaccinosis* in 1884, in which he wrote that "vaccination is a homeoprophylactic pathogenic measure: a disease is provoked to prevent a similar one—cowpox to prevent human smallpox... as in vaccinating a person we are making him ill, we are giving him vaccinosis", He had understood that the principle of artificial immunization was consonant with the law of sympathy—*similia similibus curantur*—that is also at the basis of homeopathic thought. The idea was that the vaccinations prevent a disease by causing it in a milder form, thus immunizing the organism against the effects of the natural agent. Some homeopaths even accused Pasteur of having stolen from homeopathy the method of attenuation by serial cultivation of the pathogenic agents with which he obtained his "vaccines".

The position of Compton Burnett did not prevail. John Le Gay Brereton, another influential British homeopath, declared in the same years: "I would prefer being shot rather than a relative of mine be vaccinated". Those who were at the time against vaccination, namely, the anti-smallpox vaccine (the only one existing, and the production of which was greatly contaminated) had good arguments not to be vaccinated—on the individual level but not on the statistical one: contracting smallpox naturally implied a risk of death that was much greater than the risks from inoculation of animal or human pox matter containing all sorts of other pathogens.

It is a fact that the idea of artificial immunization has its origin in magic, as Compton Burnett had understood, just as it is true that the first vaccinations were anything but safe. When the phenomenon found a scientific explanation that allowed improving the method of production and safety, homeopaths and heterodox doctors refused the vaccines; this is glaring evidence of the superstitious and fideistic nature of the so-called alternative medicines, starting from homeopathy.

Understandably, today magic thought is at the origin of the distorted perceptions of risk in the cases of vaccinations. Andrea Grignolio's book is in this sense original and very useful. It is original, considering that it is the first book that tackles the problem of the social resistance to vaccinations looking at the neurocognitive bases of those misleading perceptions of risk which induce parents not to vaccinate their children against potentially fatal diseases and it is useful because, in the light of the psychological explanations and some studies on the different efficacy of communication strategies, it suggests how public communication should be improved to intercept and orient the public towards rational choices, especially those who are undecided, not so much because they have not understood the usefulness of vaccinations but due to psychological resistance due to the pressure and disinformation typical of some subcultural contexts.

History of Medicine and Bioethics
Unit, Museum of History of
Medicine, Sapienza University of
Rome
Rome, Italy

Department of Molecular Medicine,
Sapienza University of Rome
Rome, Italy

Social Sciences and Humanities,
Cultural Heritage Department,
National Research Council
Rome, Italy

Gilberto Corbellini

# Acknowledgements

Before the acknowledgements, a few words about the title (the original Italian title was *Who is afraid of the vaccines?* [Chi ha paura dei vaccini?]). A few months ago, as I was reflecting on how to structure a book to explain to myself, and perhaps to others, why educated and intelligent people put their lives and those of their children at risk by refusing vaccinations, I happened to see again *Who's afraid of Virginia Woolf?*, an excellent film with a couple (on the set and in real life) of actors, Liz Taylor and Richard Burton, based on the play by Edward Albee and directed in 1966 by the great US director Mike Nichols—who also directed films like *The graduate* (1967) and *Closer* (2004). The film tells the story of a mature and affluent bourgeois couple who start out on a self-destructive path, fuelled by harsh discussions on the impossibility of an authentic professional and existential fulfilment. Against the background of this fierce verbal hand-to-hand combat, in an alternation of falsehoods and truths, there appear various Shakespearian shadows: the death, perhaps imaginary, of a child; the dialogues with a young naïve but sensible couple; and a series of irrational fears. These shadows are childishly exorcised by the nursery rhyme of the three little pigs which gives its title to the film—*Who's afraid of the Big Bad Wolf?*, which the couple occasionally sing to evoke not only the big bad wolf which hovers in their existence but also the English writer Virginia Woolf, who committed suicide due to a great psychic imbalance. As it will emerge, some of these topics (socio-economic affluence, the irrationality of the choices and some self-destructive attitudes potentially harmful for children) are present in the book, more or less between the lines.

This book owes a great deal to many people, directly and indirectly. Gilberto Corbellini has been and is much more than a teacher, from the times of my thesis which had a chapter on immunology. I owe to him many of the ideas that form the structural axis of the book. I owe Alfred I. Tauber my

A. Grignolio, *Vaccines: Are they Worth a Shot?*, https://doi.org/10.1007/978-3-319-68106-1

"long reasoning", still in progress, on the history and philosophy of immunology. From Michel Morange, I have learned the importance of a scientist's gaze on the history of biomedical sciences. To Claudio Franceschi, his ideas and his affection, I am particularly in debt because he showed me that in science not only the data and methods are important but also the *vision*. Lastly, I have an enormous debt to Elena Cattaneo: before meeting her I knew—from a theoretical point of view—that a great scientist is one outside the laboratory as well, but with her I had tangible proof of this.

This book, like every book, has meant many hours of work taken away from my family, hours that Francesca had to make up with little Vittoria, but she did it with affection and participation. Without her help, I could never have written it.

Over the past few years, I have had the fortune to read and measure myself up to studies by scientists whom only in time have I realized are of capital importance, some of whom have read and commented on parts of this book, and I would like to thank them here: Carlo M. Croce, Alberto Mantovani, Luca Pani, Rino Rappuoli. It is almost pointless to specify that any errors in the book are mine, and mine alone.

Part of the research for this book was done thanks to the award of a grant, *LE STUDIUM, Biopharmaceuticals Programme*, on the history of vaccination and serotherapy, at the French university of Tours François-Rabelais.

In the light of the arguments which in general fuel the debates on vaccines, I would, in the last place, like to state the absence of any form whatsoever of conflict of interest on my part.

# Bibliography

Aasheim, V. *et al.* (2012), *Associations Between Advanced Maternal Age and Psychological Distress in Primiparous Women, From Early Pregnancy To 18 Months Postpartum*, "BJOG", 119 (9), pp. 1108–16.

Aasheim, V. *et al.* (2014), *Satisfaction With Life During Pregnancy and Early Motherhood in First-Time Mothers of Advanced Age: A Population-Based Longitudinal Study*, "BMC Pregnancy Childbirth", 14, 86.

Abhyankar, P., D.B. O'Connor and R. Lawton (2008), *The Role of Message Framing in Promoting MMR Vaccination: Evidence of A Loss-Frame Advantage*, "Psychol Health Med", 13 (1), pp. 1–16.

Afzal, M.A. *et al.* (2006), *Absence of Detectable Measles Virus Genome Sequence in Blood of Autistic Children Who Have Had Their MMR Vaccination During the Routine Childhood Immunization Schedule of UK*, "Journal of Medical Virology", 78(5), pp. 623–30.

Albert, M., K.G. Ostheimer and J.G. Breman (2001), *The Last Smallpox Epidemic in Boston and The Vaccination Controversy*, "The New England Journal of Medicine", p. 344.

Amante D.J., Hogan T.P., *et al.* (2015), *Access to Care and Use of the Internet to Search for Health Information: Results From the US National Health Interview Survey*, "Journal of Medical Internet Research", 17 (4), e106.

Anderberg, D., A. Chevalier e J. Wadsworth (2011), *Anatomy of a Health Scare: Education, Income and the MMR Controversy in the UK*, "Journal of Health Economics", 30 (3), pp. 515–30.

Anderson, M. (2015), *5 facts about vaccines in the U.S.*, Pew research Center, July 17, 2015 (https://goo.gl/5GXYbj)

Andrews, N. *et al.* (2004), *Thimerosal Exposure in Infants and Developmental Disorders: A Retrospective Cohort Study in the United Kingdom Does Not Support a Causal Association*, "Pediatrics", 114 (3), pp. 584–91.

© Springer International Publishing AG, part of Springer Nature 2018

A. Grignolio, *Vaccines: Are they Worth a Shot?*, https://doi.org/10.1007/978-3-319-68106-1

Arenz, S. *et al.* (2003), *Der Masernausbruch in Coburg: Was lässt sich daraus lernen? Dtsch Arztebl International*, 100 (49), A-3245 (I used the data shown in hte artilce in English by Ernst, 2011).

Armitage, C.J. and M. Conner (2000), *Social Cognition Models and Health Behaviour: A Structured Review*, "Psychology & Health", 15 (2), pp. 173–89.

Aronson, S.M. e L. Newman (2002), *God Have Mercy on This House: Being a Brief Chronicle of Smallpox in Colonial New England*, in *Smallpox in the Americas 1492 to 1815: Contagion and Controversy*, Brown University, Exhibition at the John Carter at Brown Library, News Service, http://tinyurl.com/goyxton.

Baggs, J. *et al* (2011), *The Vaccine Safety Datalink: A Model for Monitoring Immunization Safety*, "Pediatrics", 127 Suppl 1, pp. S45–53.

Baird, G. *et al.* (2008), *Measles Vaccination and Antibody Response in Autism Spectrum Disorders*, "Archive Disease in Childhood", October, 93(10), pp. 832–37.

Baker, J. (2003), *The Pertussis Vaccine Controversy in Great Britain, 1974-1986*, "Vaccine", 21, pp. 4003–4011.

Baker, J. (2008), *Mercury, Vaccines, and Autism: One Controversy, Three Histories*, "American Journal of Public Health", 98(2), pp. 244–53.

Baker JP, Katz SL, Childhood vaccine development: an overview. Pediatr Res. 2004 Feb;55(2):347–56. Epub 2003 Nov 19.

Ball, L.K., G. Evans. and A. Bostrom (1998), *Risky Business: Challenges in Vaccine Risk Communication*, "Pediatrics", 101 (3 Pt 1), pp. 453–58.

Bandolier, *Independent Evidence-Based Thinking About Health Care*, Oxford University [authors not mentioned], "Extra Number on MMR Vaccination and Autism", April 2005, pp. 1–12.

Bates, T. (2011), *MMR Scare. In the Wake of Wakefield*, "BMJ", 342, p. d806.

Battistella, M. *et al.* (2013), *Vaccines and Autism: A Myth to Debunk?*, "Igiene e Sanità Pubblica", 69 (5), pp. 585–96.

Batzing-Feigenbaum, J. *et al.* (2010), *Spotlight on Measles 2010: Preliminary Report of An Ongoing Measles Outbreak in A Subpopulation with Low Vaccination Coverage in Berlin, Germany, January-March 2010*, "Euro Surveill", 15 (13).

Bauer, M. (1995), *Resistance to New Technology: Nuclear Power, Information Technology and Biotechnology*, Cambridge University Press, Cambridge, New York.

Bayrampour, H. *et al.* (2012), *Advanced Maternal Age and Risk Perception: A Qualitative Study*, "BMC Pregnancy and Childbirth", 12 (1), pp. 1–13.

Beaujouan, É., Sobotka, T. (2017), *Vienna Institute Of Demography. Late Motherhood In Low-Fertility Countries: Reproductive Intentions, Trends And Consequences.* Vienna Institute of Demography, Austrian Academy of Sciences (https://goo.gl/C9iqoC)

Beccaria, G. e A. Grignolio (2014), *Scienza & Democrazia. Come la ricerca demolisce i nostri pregiudizi e può migliorarci la vita*, Edizione La Stampa/40K, Torino.

Behbehani, A.M. (1983), *The Smallpox Story: Life and Death of an Old Disease*, "Microbiology Review", 47(4), pp. 455–509.

Bellavite, P., et al. (2005), *Immunology and Homeopathy. 1. Historical Background.* "Evidence-based Complementary and Alternative Medicine". 2(4): p. 441–452.

Benedetti, F. (2014), *Placebo Effects: Understanding the Mechanisms in Health and Disease*, Oxford University Press.

Berezow, A. (2017). *The Perfect American Storm: Incivility, Anti-Intellectualism, Tribalism.* The American Council on Science and Health, February 7, 2017. (https://goo.gl/Q2VTbM)

Berkes, E.A. (2003), *Anaphylactic and Anaphylactoid Reactions to Aspirin and Other NSAIDS*, "Clinical Reviews in Allergy & Immunology", 24 (2), pp. 137–48.

Bernsen, R.M. *et al.* (2006), *Early Life Circumstances and Atopic Disorders in Childhood*, "Clin Exp Allergy", 36 (7), pp. 858–65.

Bessi, A. *et al.* (2015), *Science vs Conspiracy: Collective Narratives in the Age of Misinformation*, "PLoS ONE", 10(2), e0118093.

Betsch C., Brewer N.T. et al. (2012), *Opportunities and challenges of Web 2.0 for vaccination decisions*, "Vaccine", 30, pp. 3727–3733

Biasucci, G. *et al.* (2008), *Cesarean Delivery May Affect the Early Biodiversity of Intestinal Bacteria*, "Journal of Nutrition", 138 (9), pp. 1796S–1800S.

Billari F.C., Goisis A. et al. (2011), *Social age deadlines for the childbearing of women and men*, "Hum Reprod", 26 (3), pp. 616–622.

Blanchflower, D.G. and A.J. Oswald (2008), *Is Well-Being U-Shaped Over the Life Cycle?*, "Social Science & Medicine", 66 (8), pp. 1733–49.

Blancke, S. *et al.* (2015), *Fatal Attraction: The Intuitive Appeal of GMO Opposition*, "Trends in Plant Science", 20(7), pp. 414–18.

Blendon R.J., Benson J.M *et al.* (2014), *Public Trust in Physicians – U.S. Medicine in International Perspective*, "New England Journal of Medicine", 371 (17), pp. 1570–1572.

Blumberg, S.J. *et al.* (2013), *Changes in Prevalence of Parent-Reported Autism Spectrum Disorder in School-Aged US Children: 2007 to 2011–2012*, "National Health Statistics Report", (65), pp. 1-11.

Blume, S. (2006), *Anti-Vaccination Movements and Their Interpretations*, "Social Science & Medicine", 62 (3), pp. 628–42.

Bradford W.D., Mandich A. (2015), *Some state vaccination laws contribute to greater exemption rates and disease outbreaks in the United States*, "Health Aff."; 34 (8), pp. 1383–1390.

Bray, I., D. Gunnell. and G. Davey Smith (2006), *Advanced Paternal Age: How Old Is Too Old?*, "Journal of Epidemiology & Community Health", 60 (10), pp. 851–53.

Brimnes, N. (2004), *Variolation, Vaccination and Popular Resistance in Early Colonial South India*, "Medical History", 48(2), pp. 199–228.

Broadbent, J. (2017). *Academic evidence, policy and practice.* "Public Money & Management" 37(4): 233–236.

Broderick, M.P. *et al.* (2015), *Effect of Multiple, Simultaneous Vaccines on Polio Seroresponse and Associated Health Outcomes*, "Vaccine", 33(24), pp. 2842–48.

Brown, E. (2011), *'Pox parties': Coming to a mailbox near you?*, "Los Angeles Times", Nov. 04, 2011.

Brown K.F., Long S.J., et al., (2012), *UK parents' decision-making about measles-mumps-rubella (MMR) vaccine 10 years after the MMR-autism controversy: A qualitative analysis*, "Vaccine", 30 (10). pp. 1855–1864.

Bucci, E. (2015), *Cattivi Scienziati. La frode nella ricerca scientifica*, Add Editore, Torino.

Buck, C. (2003), *Smallpox Inoculation. Should We Credit Chinese Medicine?*, "Complementary Therapies in Medicine", 11(3), pp. 201–202.

Burioni, R. (2016), *Il vaccino non è un'opinione*. Milano, Mondadori.

Burnett, J.C. (1884), *Vaccinosis and Its Cure by Thuja; With Remarks On Homeoprophylaxis*, Homoeopathic Publishing Co., London

Busse, J.W., Morgan, L. *et al.* (2005), *Chiropractic antivaccination arguments*, "J Manipulative Physiol Ther", 28, pp. 367–73.

Byford, J. (2011), *Conspiracy Theories: A Critical Introduction*, Palgrave Macmillan, London, New York.

Calvert N, Ashton JR, Garnett E., Mumps outbreak in private schools: public health lessons for the post-Wakefield era. Lancet. 2013 May 11;381(9878):1625–6.

Capocci, M., Corbellini G. (2014), *Le cellule della speranza: il caso Stamina tra inganno e scienza*, Codice edizioni, Torino.

Carolan, M. (2009), *Towards Understanding the Concept of Risk for Pregnant Women: Some Nursing and Midwifery Implications*, "Journal of Clinical Nursing", 18(5), pp. 652–58.

Carolan M. and S. Nelson (2007), *First Mothering Over 35 Years: Questioning the Association of Maternal Age and Pregnancy Risk*, "Health Care for Women International", 28(6), pp. 534–55.

Casiday R. *et al.* (2006), *A survey of UK parental attitudes to the MMR vaccine and trust in medical authority.* "Vaccine", 24 (2), pp. 177–184.

Casiday, R.E. (2007), *Children's Health and the Social Theory of Risk: Insights From the British Measles, Mumps and Rubella (MMR) Controversy*, "Social Science & Medicine" 65(5), pp. 1059–70.

Cassell, M.M. *et al.* (2006), *Risk Compensation: The Achilles' Heel of Innovations in HIV Prevention?*, "British Medical Journal", 332 (7541), pp. 605–607.

Cattaneo, E., De Falco, J., Grignolio, A. (2016), *Ogni giorno. Tra scienza e politica.* Milano, Mondadori.

Cha A.E. (2016), *7 things about vaccines and autism that the movie 'Vaxxed' won't tell you*, "The Washington Post", May 25, 2016 (https://goo.gl/WbTd4R)

Chesworth A. (2005) *Tom Cruise, Scientology Bash Psychiatry; APA Fires Back*, "Skeptical Inquirer", 2005;29.5:8–11.

Chow, Y.K.M, Danchin *et al.* (2017), *Parental attitudes, beliefs, behaviours and concerns towards childhood vaccinations in Australia: A national online survey*, "Australian Family Physician", 46 (3), pp. 145–151.

Cillizza, C. (2016), *Donald Trump's post-truth campaign and what it says about the dismal state of US politics*, "The Independent", May 10th 2016, June 19th 2017 (https://goo.gl/znPsmw)

Conforti, M., G. Corbellini e G. Gazzaniga (2012), *Dalla cura alla scienza. Malattia, salute e società nel mondo occidentale*, Milano, EncycloMedia.

Corbellini, G. (2011), *Scienza quindi democrazia*, Einaudi, Torino.

Corbellini, G. (2009), *Perché gli scienziati non sono pericolosi : scienza, etica, e politica*, Milano, Longanesi.

Corbellini, G. (2013), *Scienza*, Bollati Boringhieri, Torino.

Covello, V.T., D. von Winterfeldt and P. Slovic (1986), *Communicating Scientific Information About Health and Environmental Risks: Problems and Opportunities from a Social and Behavioral Perspective*, in V.T. Covello, A. Moghissi e V. Uppulori, *Uncertainties in Risk Assessment and Risk Management*, Plenum Press, New York, p. 221–239.

Covello, V.T. and P.M. Sandman (2001), *Risk Communication: Evolution and Revolution*, in W.A. (ed) *Solutions to An Environment in Peril*, John Hopkins University Press, Baltimora, pp. 164–78.

Crimmins, E.M., S.H. Preston and B.C. Cohen (2011), *Explaining Divergent Levels of Longevity in High-Income Countries*, in *Panel on Understanding Divergent Trends in Longevity in High-Income Countries*, National Research Council (US), Vol. 37, National Academies Press, Washington D.C., pp. 791–93.

D'Souza, Y., E. Fombonne and B.J. Ward (2006), *No Evidence of Persisting Measles Virus in Peripheral Blood Mononuclear Cells From Children With Autism Spectrum Disorder*, "Pediatrics", 118(4), pp. 1664–75

Daguet, A. and H. Watier (2011), *2nd Charles Richet and Jules Hericourt Workshop: Therapeutic Antibodies And Anaphylaxis; May 31–June 1, 2011, Tours, France*, "MAbs", 3(5), pp. 417–21.

Daguet, A. and H. Watier (2012), *Serotherapy, Among Therapeutic Innovations and Scientific Progress in the Late 19th And 20th Centuries*, "La Revue du praticien", 62 (8), pp. 1177–81.

Dales, L., S.J. Hammer and N.J. Smith (2001), *Time Trends in Autism and in MMR Immunization Coverage in California*, "JAMA", March, 7, 285(9), pp. 1183–85.

Davidovitch, N. (2004), *Homeopathy and Anti-Vaccinationism at the Turn of the Twentieth Century*, in R.D. Johnston (ed), *The Politics of Healing: Histories of Alternative Medicine in Twentieth-Century North America*, Routledge, New York, p. 11–28.

Davis, C. (1978), *Variolation in the Rajasthan Desert* ,"Indian Journal of Public Health", 22(1), pp. 134–40.

Debley, J.S. *et al.* (2005), *Childhood Asthma Hospitalization Risk After Cesarean Delivery in Former Term and Premature Infants*, "Annals of Allergy, Asthma & Immunology", 94 (2), pp. 228–33.

Debord, G. (1967), *Commentari sulla società dello spettacolo e La società dello spettacolo*. Milano, Sugarco, 1990 (original edition: *La Société du spectacle*, Paris, éditions Buchet/Chastel).

Deer, B. (2004), *Revealed: MMR Research Scandal*, "The Sunday Times", 22 February.

Deer, B. (2011a), *How the Case against the MMR Vaccine Was Fixed*, "BMJ", 342, c5347.

Deer, B. (2011b), *How the Vaccine Crisis Was Meant to Make Money*, "BMJ", 342.

Deisher, T.A. *et al.* (2015), *Epidemiologic And Molecular Relationship Between Vaccine Manufacture and Autism Spectrum Disorder Prevalence*, "Issues in Law & Medicine", 30 (1), pp. 47–70.

DeStefano F, Thompson WW., MMR vaccine and autism: an update of the scientific evidence. Expert Rev Vaccines. 2004 Feb;3(1):19–22.

DeStefano, F., C.S. Price and E.S. Weintraub (2013), *Increasing Exposure to Antibodystimulating Proteins and Polysaccharides in Vaccines is Not Associated With Risk of Autism*, "Journal of Pediatrics", August 163(2), p. 5617.

Diamond, J.M. (1998), *Armi, acciaio e malattie*, Einaudi, Torino (original edition *Guns, Germs, and Steel: The Fates of Human Societies*, 1998).

Diel, R. *et al.* (2014), *Costs of Tuberculosis Disease in the European Union: A Systematic Analysis and Cost Calculation*, "European Respiratory Journal", 43 (2), pp. 554–65.

Dinc, G. e Y. I. Ulman (2007), *The Introduction of Variolation "A La Turca" to The West By Lady Mary Montagu And Turkey's Contribution to This*", "Vaccine", 25(21), pp. 4261–65.

Dobrovolskaya, M.V., *Upper Palaeolithic and Late Stone Age Human Diet*, "Journal of Physiological Anthropology and Applied Human Science", 2005, 24 (4), pp. 433–38.

Dominguez-Bello, M.G. *et al.* (2010), *Delivery Mode Shapes the Acquisition and Structure of the Initial Microbiota Across Multiple Body Habitats in Newborns*, "PNAS", 107 (26), pp. 11.971–75.

Douglas R.G., Samant V.B. (2017), The Vaccine Industry. In: J.L. Schwartz, A.L. Caplan (Eds.), *Vaccination Ethics and Policy. An Introduction with Readings*, MIT University Press, Cambridge, MA.

Dove, A. (2005), *Maurice Hilleman*, "Nature Medicine", 11(4 Suppl), S2.

Downey, L., Tyree, P.T. *et al.* (2010), *Pediatric vaccination and vaccine-preventable disease acquisition: Associations with care by complementary and alternative medicine providers*, "Matern Child Health J." 14(6): pp. 922–30.

Drezner, D.W. (2016), *Why the post-truth political era might be around for a while*, "The Washington Post", June 16th 2016, June 19th 2017 (https://goo.gl/4sdej2)

Dube, E., Vivion, M. et al. (2013), *How do Midwives and Physicians Discuss Childhood Vaccination with Parents?*, "J Clin Med", 2 (4), 242–59.

Dudley, R. (2000), *Evolutionary Origins of Human Alcoholism in Primate Frugivory*, "The Quarterly Review of Biology", 75(1), pp. 3–15.

Duffell E, Attitudes of parents towards measles and immunisation after a measles outbreak in an anthroposophical community. J Epidemiol Community Health. 2001 Sep;55(9):685–6.

Durbach, N. (2000). *They Might As Well Brand Us: Working Class Resistance to Compulsory Vaccination in Victorian England*, "The Society for the Social History of Medicine", 13, pp. 45–62.

Emanuel, E.J. and C. Grady (2008), *Four Paradigms of Clinical Research and Research Oversight*, in *The Oxford Textbook of Clinical Research Ethics*, E.J. Emanuel *et al.*, Oxford University Press, Oxford, New York, pp. 222–30.

Ernst, E. (1995), *Homoeopaths and Chiropractors Are Sceptical About Immunisation*, "BMJ" 311(7008), p. 811.

Ernst, E. (2001), *Rise in Popularity of Complementary and Alternative Medicine: Reasons and Consequences for Vaccination*, "Vaccine", 20 suppl. 1, S90–93, discussion S89.

Ernst, E. (2011), *Anthroposophy: A Risk Factor for Noncompliance with Measles Immunization*, "The Pediatric Infectious Disease Journal", 30(3), pp. 187–89.

Escritt, T. (2017), *German Kindergartens to Name Parents Who Refuse Vaccine Advice Europe is experiencing a spike in disease thanks to a drop in immunization numbers.* "Scientific American", May 26, 2017 (https://goo.gl/XnpnGr).

Ethgen O., Baron-Papillon F., Cornier M. (2016), *How much money is spent on vaccines across Western European countries?*, "Human Vaccines & Immunotherapeutics", 12 (8), pp. 2038–2045.

Evans CF, Davtyan H, Petrushina I *et al.*, Epitope-based DNA vaccine for Alzheimer's disease: translational study in macaques. Alzheimers Dement. 2014 May;10 (3):284–95.

Finucane, M.L. (2002), *Mad Cows, Mad Corn and Mad Communities: The Role of Socio-Cultural Factors in the Perceived Risk of Genetically-Modified Food*, "Proceedings of the Nutrition Society", 61(1), pp. 31–37.

Flower, D.R. (2008), *Variolation in History*, in D. R. Flower, *Bioinformatics for Vaccinology*, Wiley-Blackwell, Oxford, pp. 5, 6.

Flynn, J.R. (2013), *Osa pensare: venti concetti per capire criticamente e apprezzare la modernità*. Mondadori università, Milano (original edition *How to Improve Your Mind Twenty Keys to Unlock the Modern World*, 2012).

Fontanella, C.A. *et al.* (2015), *Widening Rural-Urban Disparities in Youth Suicides, United States, 1996-2010*, "JAMA Pediatrics", 169 (5), pp. 466–73.

Franceschi, C., M. Bonafè e S. Valensin (2000), *Human Immunosenescence: The Prevailing of Innate Immunity, the Failing of Clonotypic Immunity, and the Filling of Immunological Space*, "Vaccine", 18 (16), pp. 1717–20.

Freedland, J. (2016), *Post-truth politicians such as Donald Trump and Boris Johnson are no joke*, "The Guardian", May 13th 2016, June 19th 2017 (https://goo.gl/CWtgjS)

Gadad, B.S. *et al.* (2015), *Administration of Thimerosal-Containing Vaccines to Infant Rhesus Macaques Does Not Result in Autism-Like Behavior Or Neuropathology*, "Proceedings of the National Academy of Sciences", 112 (40), pp. 12.498-503.

Galanakis, E. *et al.* (2013), *Ethics of Mandatory Vaccination for Healthcare Workers*, "Euro Surveill", 18 (45), p. 20.627.

Galanakis, E. *et al.* (2014), *The Issue of Mandatory Vaccination for Healthcare Workers in Europe*, Expert Rev Vaccines, 13 (2), pp. 277–83.

Galazka, A. and S. Dittmann (2000*), Implications of the Diphtheria Epidemic in the Former Soviet Union for Immunization Programs*, Journal of Infectious Diseases, 181 (Supplement 1), S244–S248.

Galeotti, F. *et al.* (2013), *Risk of Guillain-Barre Syndrome after 2010-2011 Influenza Vaccination*, "European Journal of Epidemiology", 2013, 28 (5), pp. 433–44.

Gallant, D. M., Vollman, A. R. *et al.* (2009), *Influenza vaccination by registered nurses: a personal decision*, "Can J Infect Control", 24 (1), 18–22.

Gangarosa, E.J. *et al.* (1998), *Impact of Anti-Vaccine Movements on Pertussis Control: The Untold Story*, "Lancet", 351, pp. 356–61.

Gentilcore, D. (2006). *Medical Charlatanism in Early Modern Italy*, Oxford University Press, Oxford, New York.

Gentile, I. *et al.* (2013), *Response to Measlesmumpsrubella Vaccine in Children with Autism Spectrum Disorders*, "Vivo MayJun", 27(3), p. 37.782.

Ghianni, T., *Swapping chicken pox-infected lollipops illegal*, "Reuters Health News", Nov 12, 2011.

Gigerenzer, G. (1996), *On Narrow Norms and Vague Heuristics: A Reply to Kahneman and Tversky*, "Psychological Review", 103(3), pp. 592–96.

Gigerenzer, G. (2009), *Decisioni intuitive: quando si sceglie senza pensarci troppo*, Cortina, Milano (original edition, *Gut Feelings: The Intelligence of the Unconscious*, 2007).

Gigerenzer, G. (2015), *Imparare a rischiare: come prendere decisioni giuste*, Cortina, Milano (original edition: *Risk Savvy: How to Make Good Decisions*, 2014).

Gigerenzer, G. e J.A.M. Gray (2013), *Better Doctors, Better Patients, Better Decisions: Envisioning Health Care 2020* , MIT Press, Cambridge, MA.

Ginzburg, C. (2000), *Rapporti di forza. Storia, retorica, prova*. Feltrinelli, Milano (Engl. transl.: *History, Rhetoric, and Proof (The Menahem Stern Jerusalem Lectures)*. Brandeis University Press/Historical Society of Israel, 1999).

Ginzburg, C. (2006), *Il filo e le tracce. Vero, falso, finto*. Feltrinelli, Milano (Engl. transl.: *Threads and Traces: True False Fictive*. University of California Press, 2012).

Gnadinger, M., M. Gassner and G. Bachmann (2009), *Attitudes Towards Vaccination: Users of Complementary and Alternative Medicine Versus Non-Users*, "Swiss Medical Weekly", 139 (13–14), p. 212; author's reply on p. 212.

Godlee, F., J. Smith, H. Marcovitch (2011), *Wakefield's Article Linking Mmr Vaccine and Autism Was Fraudulent*, "BMJ", 342.

Goldhaber-Fiebert JD, Lipsitch et al. (2010), *Quantifying child mortality reductions related to measles vaccination*, PLoS ONE, e13842.

Gostin, L.O. (2005). *Jacobson v Massachusetts at 100 Years: Police Power and Civil Liberties in Tension*, "American Journal of Public Health", 95(4), pp. 576–81.

Gray J.A. (1999), *Postmodern medicine*, "Lancet", 354 (9189), pp. 1550–1553.

Greenberg J., Dube E., Driedger M. (2017), *Vaccine Hesitancy: In Search of the Risk Communication Comfort Zone*, "PLoS Curr", 9.

Greenough, P.R. (1980), *Variolation and Vaccination in South Asia, c. 1700-1865: A Preliminary Note*, "Social Science & Medicine. Part D: Medical Geography", 14D (3), pp. 345–47.

Gregson, A.L., R. Edelman (2003), *Does Antigenic Overload Exist? The Role of Multiple Immunizations in Infants*, "Immunology and Allergy Clinics of North America" 23 (4), pp. 649–64.

Grignolio, A. (2010), (ed. by), *Immunology Today. Three Historical Perspectives Under Three Theoretical Horizons*, Bononia Univeristy Press, Bologna.

Grignolio, A. (2015), *L'influenza di alcune idee relativiste sull'antiscientismo*. In M. Cappato (ed.), *Fra scienza e politica. Il difficile cammino della libertà di ricerca*, Carocci editore, Rome, pp. 125–37.

Grignolio A. (2017), *Post-verità, vaccini, democrazia*, "Future of Science and Ethics", 2, pp. 75–88.

Grignolio, A. , Franceschi C. (2012), *History of Research into Ageing/Senescence*, in WF Bynum (ed), eLS. John Wiley & Sons, Ltd, Chichester.

Grignolio, A., Mishto M. *et al.* (2014), *Towards a Liquid Self: How Time, Geography, and Life Experiences Reshape the Biological Identity*, "Frontiers in Immunology", 5, p. 153.

Grignolio A., Cattaneo E. (2014), *The story of Carmine Vona"*. In C.L. Mummery, B.A.J. Roelen, A. van de Stolpe, H. Clevers (Eds), *Stem Cells: Scientific Facts and Fiction*, Elsevier, 2nd edition, London, pp. 310–312.

Grmek, M.D. (1985), *Le malattie all'alba della civiltà occidentale*, Il Mulino, Bologna (original edition *Les maladies à l'aube de la civilisation occidentale*, 1983).

Gronlund, M.M. *et al.* (1999), *Fecal Microflora in Healthy Infants Born by Different Methods of Delivery: Permanent Changes in Intestinal Flora After Cesarean Delivery*, "Journal of Pediatric Gastroenterology and Nutrition", 28 (1), pp. 19–25.

Gross, C.P., Sepkowitz, K.A. (1998), *The Myth of the Medical Breakthrough: Smallpox, Vaccination, and Jenner Reconsidered*, "International Journal of Infectious Diseases", 3(1), pp. 54–60.

Gruber, C. *et al.* (2008), *Early Atopic Disease and Early Childhood Immunization – Is There A Link?*, "Allergy", 63 (11), pp. 1464–72.

Haidt, J. (2013), *Menti tribali: perché le brave persone si dividono su politica e religione*, Codice edizioni, Torino (original edition *The Righteous Mind: Why Good People Are Divided by Politics and Religion*, 2012).

Hammarsten, J. F., Tattersall, W. *et al.* (1979), *Who discovered smallpox vaccination? Edward Jenner or Benjamin Jesty?*, "Trans Am Clin Climatol Assoc", 90, 44–55.

Hanratty, B. *et al.* (2000), *UK Measles Outbreak In Non-Immune Anthroposophic Communities: The Implications for The Elimination of Measles from Europe*, "Epidemiol Infect", 125 (2), pp. 377–83.

Hansen, S.N., D.E. Schendel e E.T. Parner (2015), *Explaining the Increase in the Prevalence of Autism Spectrum Disorders: The Proportion Attributable to Changes in Reporting Practices*, "JAMA Pediatrics", 169 (1), pp. 56–62.

Haverkate, M. *et al.* (2012). *Mandatory and Recommended Vaccination in the EU, Iceland and Norway: Results of the Venice 2010 Survey on the Ways of Implementing National Vaccination Programmes*, Euro Surveill, 17(22).

Heck Hd, Casanova M, The implausibility of leukemia induction by formaldehyde: a critical review of the biological evidence on distant-site toxicity. Regul Toxicol Pharmacol. 2004 Oct;40(2):92–106.

Heidinger, B.J. *et al.* (2016), *Parental Age Influences Offspring Telomere Loss*, "Functional Ecology", Jan.

Hendrix, K.S. *et al.* (2014), *Vaccine Message Framing and Parents' Intent to Immunize Their Infants for MMR*, "Pediatrics", 134 (3), e675–683.

Herbert, E.W. (1975), *Smallpox Inoculation in Africa*, "The Journal of African History", 16 (4), pp. 539–59.

Hilton, S. *et al.* (2006), *Combined Vaccines Are Like a Sudden Onslaught to the Body's Immune System: Parental Concerns About Vaccine "Overload" And "Immune-Vulnerability"*, "Vaccine", 24(20), pp. 4321–27.

Hobson-West P. (2007), *'Trusting blindly can be the biggest risk of all': organized resistance to childhood vaccination in the UK*, "Sociology of Health and Illness", 29(2), pp. 198–215.

Hogg, M.A. e D.L. Blaylock (2011), *Extremism and the Psychology of Uncertainty*, Wiley-Blackwell, Malden, MA.

Honda, H., Y. Shimizu e M. Rutter (2005), *No Effect of MMR Withdrawal on the Incidence of Autism: A Total Population Study*, "Journal of Child Psychology Psychiatry", 46(6), pp. 572–79.

Horne, Z. *et al.* (2015), *Countering Antivaccination Attitudes*, "Proceedings of the National Academy of Sciences", 112 (33), pp. 10.321–24.

Hornig, M. *et al.* (2008), *Lack of Association Between Measles Virus Vaccine and Autism With Enteropathy: A Case-Control Study*, "PLoS One", 4,3(9), e3140.

Hough-Telford, C., Kimberlin, D. W. et al. (2016). *Vaccine Delays, Refusals, and Patient Dismissals: A Survey of Pediatricians*, "Pediatrics", 138(3).

Huth, E. (2006), *Quantitative Evidence for Judgments on the Efficacy of Inoculation for the Prevention of Smallpox: England and New England in the 1700s*, "Journal of the Royal Society of Medicine", 99(5), pp. 262–66.

Iizuka, M. *et al.* (2000), *Immunohistochemical Analysis of the Distribution of Measles Related Antigen in the Intestinal Mucosa in Inflammatory Bowel Disease*, "Gut", 46 (2), pp. 163–69.

Iqbal, S. *et al.* (2013), *Number of Antigens in Early Childhood Vaccines and Neuropsychological Outcomes at Age 7-10 Years*, "Pharmacoepidemiology and Drug Safety", December, 22(12), p. 126.370.

Jain A, Marshall J et al., Autism occurrence by MMR vaccine status among US children with older siblings with and without autism. JAMA. 2015 Apr 21;313 (15):1534–40.

Jervis, G. (2014), *Contro il sentito dire. Psicoanalisi, psichiatria e politica*, Bollati Boringhieri, Torino.

Jick, H., J.A. Kaye e C. Black (2003), *Changes in Risk of Autism in the UK for Birth Cohorts 1990-1998*, "Epidemiology", 14(5), pp. 630–32.

Jick, H., D.P Chamberlin and K.W. Hagberg (2009), *The Origin and Spread of a Mumps Epidemic: United Kingdom, 2003-2006*, "Epidemiology", 20, pp. 656–61.

Johnson, N.P. and J. Mueller (2002), *Updating the Accounts: Global Mortality of the 1918-1920 "Spanish" Influenza Pandemic*, "Bulletin of the History of Medicine", 76 (1), pp. 105–15.

Jolley, D. and K.M. Douglas (2013), *The Social Consequences of Conspiracism: Exposure to Conspiracy Theories Decreases Intentions to Engage in Politics and to Reduce one's Carbon Footprint*, "British Journal of Psychology", 105 (1), pp. 35–56.

Jones AM, *et al.* (2012), *Parents' source of vaccine information and impact on vaccine attitudes, beliefs and nonmedical exemptions*, "Adv Prev Med", pp. 932741.

Kahan, D.M. (2010), *Fixing the Communications Failure*, "Nature", 463, pp. 296–97.

Kahan, D.M. (2012), *Cultural Cognition As a Conception of the Cultural Theory of Risk*, in *Handbook of Risk Theory Epistemology, Decision Theory, Ethics, and Social Implications of Risk*, S. Roeser, B.V. Springer, "Science+Business Media", New York, pp. 725–59.

Kahan, D.M. (2014), *Vaccine Risk Perceptions and Ad Hoc Risk Communication: An Empirical Assessment, CCP Risk Perception Studies Report No. 17*, "Yale Law & Economics Research Paper", 491, pp. 1–82.

Kahan, D.M. *et al.* (2009), *Cultural Cognition of the Risks and Benefits of Nanotechnology*, "Nature Nanotechnology", 4(2), pp. 87–91.

Kahan, D.M., H. Jenkins-Smith and D. Braman (2011), *Cultural Cognition of Scientific Consensus*, "Journal of Risk Research", 14, pp. 147–74.

Kahan, D.M. *et al.* (2012), *The Polarizing Impact of Science Literacy and Numeracy on Perceived Climate Change Risks*, "Nature Climate Change", 2 (10), pp. 732–35.

Kahneman, D. (2012). *Pensieri lenti e veloci*, Mondadori, Milano (original edition, *Thinking, Fast And Slow*, 2011).

Kahneman, D. and A. Tversky (1996), *On the Reality of Cognitive Illusions*, "Psychology Review", 103(3), pp. 582–91, discussion on p. 592–6.

Kata, A. (2010), *A Postmodern Pandora's Box: Anti-Vaccination Misinformation on the Internet*, "Vaccine", 28 (7), pp. 1709–16.

Kaufman M. (1967), *The American Anti-Vaccinationists and Their Arguments*, "Bulletin of the History of Medicine", September-October, 41(5), pp. 463–78.

Kaye, J.A., M.M. Melero-Montes and H. Jick (2001), *Mumps, Measles, and Rubella Vaccine and the Incidence of Autism Recorded by General Practitioners: A Time-Trend Analysis*, "BMJ", 322, pp. 460–63.

Kayne, S. (2006), *Samuel Hahnemann (1755-1843): the founder of modern homeopathy*. "Pharm Hist" (Lond). 36 (2 Suppl), pp. S23–6.

Keith, L.S., D.E. Jones and C.H. Chou (2002), *Aluminum Toxicokinetics Regarding Infant Diet and Vaccinations*, "Vaccine", 20 Suppl. 3, pp. S13–17.

Kelemen, D. *et al.* (2005), *Why Things Happen: Teleological Explanation in Parent-Child Conversations*, "Developmental Psychology", 41(1), pp. 251–64.

Kelemen, D. and E. Rosset (2009), *The Human Function Compunction: Teleological Explanation in Adults*, "Cognition", 111(1), pp. 138–43.

Kelemen, D., J. Rottman and R. Seston (2012), *Professional Physical Scientists Display Tenacious Teleological Tendencies: Purpose-Based Reasoning As A Cognitive Default*, "Journal Experimental Psychology", January 142(4), pp. 1074–83.

Kent, S. A. , Manca T. A. (2013), *A war over mental health professionalism: Scientology versus psychiatry*, "Ment Health Relig Cult" 17(1), pp. 1–23.

Knight, B. (2015), *Measles death in Germany prompts calls for mandatory vaccinations*, "The Guardian", 23 February, 2015.

Kriwy, P. (2011), *Similarity of Parents and Physicians in the Decision to Vaccinate Children Against Measles, Mumps And Rubella*, "International Journal of Public Health", 57(2), pp. 333–40.

Kruglanski, A.W. and D.M. Webster (1996), *Motivated Closing of the Mind: "Seizing" and "Freezing"*, "Psychology Review", 103(2), pp. 263–83.

Kuipers, R.S., J.C. Joordens and F.A Muskiet. (2012), *A Multidisciplinary Reconstruction of Palaeolithic Nutrition that Holds Promise for the Prevention and Treatment of Diseases of Civilisation*, "Nutrition Research Reviews", 25 (1), pp. 96–129.

Kuntz, M. (2017). *Science and Postmodernism: From Right-Thinking to Soft-Despotism.* "Trends in Biotechnology", 35(4), pp. 283–285.

Kuriyan A.E., Albini T.A., et al., (2017), *Vision Loss after Intravitreal Injection of Autologous "Stem Cells" for AMD*, "New England Journal of Medicine", 376 (11), pp. 1047–1053.

Kutty, P.K. *et al.* (2010), *Seroprevalence of Antibody to Mumps Virus in The US Population, 1999-2004*, "The Journal of Infection Diseases", 202 (5), pp. 667–74.

La Condamine, C.M. (1773), *Histoire de l'inoculation de la petite vérole*, Amsterdam.

La Torre, G. *et al.* (2009), *Behaviours Regarding Preventive Measures Against Pandemic H1n1 Influenza Among Italian Healthcare Workers*, October 2009, "Euro Surveill", 14 (49).

Lampinen R, Vehviläinen-Julkunen K, Kankkunen P., A review of pregnancy in women over 35 years of age. Open Nurs J. 2009 Aug 6; 3: 33–8.

Lanza F.L., F.K. Chan and E.M. Quigley (2009), *Guidelines for Prevention of Nsaid-Related Ulcer Complications*, "The American Journal of Gastroenterology", 104 (3), pp. 728–38.

Larson, H., Schulz W. (2015), *The State of Vaccine Confidence report*, The Vaccine Confidence Project - London School of Hygiene & Tropical Medicine, London (https://goo.gl/YSf2EF)

Le Couteur P. and J. Burreson (2006), *I bottoni di Napoleone: come 17 molecole hanno cambiato la storia*, Longanesi, Milano (oroiginal edition, *Napoleon's Buttons: How 17 Molecules Changed History*, 2003).

Lee, B. (2016), *Robert De Niro: 'I'm not anti-vaccine, I want safe vaccines'*, "The Guardian" 13th April 2016: https://goo.gl/R5LVa1

Leman, P.J. and M. Cinnirella (2013), *Beliefs in Conspiracy Theories and the Need for Cognitive Closure*, "Frontiers in Psychology", 4.

Lewinjan, T. (2015), *Sick Child's Father Seeks Vaccination Requirement in California*, "The New York Times" 28, 2015. (https://goo.gl/mKrASU)

Leon, D.A. *et al.* (1997), *Huge Variation in Russian Mortality Rates 1984-94: Artefact, Alcohol, Or What?*, "The Lancet", 350 (9075), pp. 383–88.

Lewandowsky, S., *et al.* (2013), *The Role of Conspiracist Ideation and Worldviews in Predicting Rejection of Science*, "PLoS ONE", 8(10), p. e75637.

Lidsky, T.I. (2014), *Is the Aluminum Hypothesis Dead?*, "Journal of Occupational and Environmental Medicine", 56(5 Suppl), pp. S73–S79.

Lorefice, L. *et al.* (2014), *Monoclonal Antibodies: A Target Therapy for Multiple Sclerosis*, "Inflammation & Allergy-Drug Targets", 13 (2), pp. 134–43.

Luthi-Carter, R. (2003), *Progress Towards a Vaccine for Huntington's Disease*, "Molecular Therapy", 7 (5 Pt 1), pp. 569–70.

Ma, B. (1995), *Variolation, Pioneer of Modern Immunology*, "Zhonghua Yi Shi Za Zhi", 25(3), pp. 139–44.

Madsen, K.M. *et al.* (2002), *MMR Vaccination And Autism. A Population-Based Follow-Up Study*, Ugeskr Laeger, 164 (49), pp. 5741–44 (I was only able to read the data and the conclusions in English of this study in Danish).

Madsen, K.M. *et al.* (2003), *Thimerosal and the Occurrence of Autism: Negative Ecological Evidence From Danish Population-Based Data*, "Pediatrics", 112 (3 Pt 1), pp. 604–606.

Majcen, S. (2016), *Evidence Based Policy Making in The European Union: The Role of the Scientific Community*, "Environmental Science and Pollution Research".

Majumder, M.S. *et al.* (2015), *Substandard Vaccination Compliance and the 2015 Measles Outbreak*, "JAMA Pediatrics", 169(5), pp. 494–95.

Mantovani, A. and M. Florianello (2016), *Immunità e vaccini. Perché è giusto proteggere la nostra salute e quella dei nostri figli*, Mondadori, Milano.

Martin M, Badalyan V, Vaccination practices among physicians and their children. Open Journal of Pediatrics 2 (2012) 228–235.

Marti M, de Cola M, *et al.*( 2017), *Assessments of global drivers of vaccine hesitancy in 2014 -- Looking beyond safety concerns*, PLoS ONE,12, e0172310.

Marx, J. (2010), *Rosen's Emergency Medicine: Concepts and Clinical Practice, 7th edition*, Mosby/Elsevier, Philadelphia, Vol. I, p. 2422.

Mason, P.H., A. Grignolio *et al.* (2015), *Hidden in Plain View: Degeneracy in Complex Systems*, "Biosystems", 128 (0), pp. 1–8.

Mather, M. (2012),*The Decline in U.S. Fertility*, Population Reference Bureau: World Population Data Sheet (https://goo.gl/n0igvh)

Matthews T.J., Hamilton B.E. (2009), Delayed childbearing: more women are having their first child later in life, NCHS data brief, no 21. Hyattsville, MD, National Center for Health Statistics.

Matthews T.J., Brady E., Hamilton B.E. (2014), First births to older women continue to rise. NCHS Data Brief, (152): pp. 1–8.

Maugh, T.H. (2005), *Obituaries. Maurice R. Hilleman, 85; Scientist Developed Many Vaccines That Saved Millions of Lives*, "Los Angeles Times", 13 April 2005.

Mazumdar, P.M.H. (1995), *Species and Specificity: An Interpretation of the History of Immunology*, Cambridge University Press, Cambridge.

McBride DL (2015), *Measles Vaccination Associated With Lower Mortality Risk From Other Childhood Infections*, J Pediatr Nurs, 30, 802–3.

McDevitt, M., P. Parks, et al. (2017). *Anti-intellectualism among US students in journalism and mass communication: A cultural perspective.* "Journalism" 0(0): 1464884917710395.

McGreevy P (2015) Not enough signatures: Vaccine opponents fall short in ballot effort. Los Angeles Times, 30 September. (https://goo.gl/63iv3j)

McNeil, M.M. *et al.* (2014), *The Vaccine Safety Datalink: Successes and Challenges Monitoring Vaccine Safety*, "Vaccine", 32 (42), pp. 5390–5398.

Merrick, J., I. Kandel and M. Morad (2004), *Trends in Autism*, "International Journal of Adolescent Medicine and Health",16(1), pp. 75–78.

Messerli, F.H. (2012), *Chocolate Consumption, Cognitive Function, and Nobel Laureates*, "New England Journal of Medicine", 367 (16), pp. 1562–1564.

Miller, D.L. and E.M. Ross (1978), *National Childhood Encephalopathy Study: An Interim Report*, "British Medical Journal", 2, pp. 992, 993.

Miller, E. *et al.* (2003), *Bacterial Infections, Immune Overload, and MMR Vaccine. Measles, Mumps, and Rubella*, "Archives of Disease in Childhood", 88(3), pp. 222–23.

Mina, M.J. *et al.* (2014), *Long-Term Measles-Induced Immunomodulation Increases Overall Childhood Infectious Disease Mortality*, "Science", 348 (6235), pp. 694–99.

Mitkus, R.J. *et al.* (2011), *Updated Aluminum Pharmacokinetics Following Infant Exposures Through Diet And Vaccination*, "Vaccine", 29 (51), pp. 9538–43.

*MMR Vaccine. Measles, Mumps, and Rubella*, "Archives of Disease in Childhood", 88 (3), pp. 222, 223.

Momigliano, A. (1985), *La storia tra medicina e retorica*, in A. Momigliano, *Tra storia e storicismo 1-24*, Nistri-Lischi Editori, Pisa, pp. 11–32.

Montana, M. *et al.* (2010), *Safety Review: Squalene and Thimerosal In Vaccines*, "Therapie", 65 (6), pp. 533–41.

Morini S. (2014), *Il Rischio. Da Pascal a Fukushima*, Bollati Boringhieri, Torino.

Moulin, A.M. (1996), *L'Aventure de la vaccination*, Paris, Fayard.

Mummery, C.L., Roelen, B.A.J., van de Stolpe, A., Clevers H. (Eds) (2014), *Stem Cells: Scientific Facts and Fiction*, Elsevier, 2nd edition, London, pp. 310–312.

Munro, G.D. and P.H. Ditto (1997), *Biased Assimilation, Attitude Polarization, and Affect in Reactions to Stereotype-Relevant Scientific Information*, "Personality and Social Psychology Bulletin", 23(6), pp. 636–53.

Munro, S. *et al.* (2007), *A Review of Health Behaviour Theories: How Useful Are These for Developing Interventions to Promote Long-Term Medication Adherence for TB And HIV/AIDS?*, "BMC Public Health", 7, p. 104.

Murch, S.H. *et al.* (2004), *Retraction of an Interpretation*, "Lancet", 363 (9411), p. 750.

Myers, G.J. *et al.* (2003), *Prenatal Methylmercury Exposure from Ocean Fish Consumption in The Seychelles Child Development Study*, "Lancet", 361(9370), pp. 1686–92.

Nagourney A (2015), *California mandates vaccines for schoolchildren*, "The New York Times", June 30th, 2015.

Namer M, Luporsi E, Gligorov J, Lokiec F, Spielmann M, L'utilisation de déodorants/antitranspirants ne constitue pas un risque de cancer du sein. Bull Cancer. 2008 Sep;95(9):871–80.

Nassar, N. *et al.* (2009), *Autism Spectrum Disorders in Young Children: Effect of Changes in Diagnostic Practices*, "International Journal of Epidemiology", 38 (5), pp. 1245–54.

Natarajan AT, Darroudi F, Bussman CJ, van Kesteren-van Leeuwen AC., Evaluation of the mutagenicity of formaldehyde in mammalian cytogenetic assays in vivo and vitro. Mutat Res. 1983 Dec;122(3–4):355–60.

Needham, J., N. Sivin and G.D. Lu (2010), *Science and Civilisation in China*, Cambridge University Press, Cambridge, Vol. 6 (original edition, 1954-1984).

Negele, K. *et al.* (2004), *Mode of Delivery and Development of Atopic Disease During the First 2 Years of Life*, "Pediatric Allergy and Immunology", 15 (1), pp. 48–54.

Nelson, M.C. and J. Rogers (1992), *The Right to Die? Anti-Vaccination Activity and the 1874 Smallpox Epidemic in Stockholm*, "Social History of Medicine", 5 December, (3), pp. 369–88.

Neu, J. and J. Rushing (2011), *Cesarean Versus Vaginal Delivery: Long-Term Infant Outcomes and the Hygiene Hypothesis*, "Clinics in Perinatology", 38 (2), pp. 321–31.

Neumayer, E. and T. Plumper (2015), *Inequalities of Income and Inequalities of Longevity: A Cross-Country Study*, "American Journal of Public Health".

Nilsen, A.B. *et al.* (2012), *Characteristics of Women Who Are Pregnant With Their First Baby at An Advanced Age*, "Acta Obstetricia Gynecologica Scandinavica", 91 (3), pp. 353–362x.

Nilsen A.B. *et al.* (2013), *Characteristics of First-Time Fathers of Advanced Age: A Norwegian Population-Based Study*, "BMC Pregnancy Childbirth", 13, p. 29.

Nyhan, B. *et al.* (2014), *Effective Messages in Vaccine Promotion: A Randomized Trial*, "Pediatrics", 133 (4), pp. e835–842.

Offit, P.A. *et al.* (2002), *Addressing Parents' Concerns: Do Multiple Vaccines Overwhelm Or Weaken The Infant's Immune System?*, "Pediatrics", 109(1), pp. 124–29.

Offit PA, Jew RK. Addressing parents' concerns: do vaccines contain harmful preservatives, adjuvants, additives, or residuals?. Pediatrics. 2003 Dec;112(6 Pt 1):1394–7.

Offit, P.A. (2005), *Why are pharmaceutical companies gradually abandoning vaccines?*, "Health Aff.", 24 (3), pp. 622–630.

Offit, P.A. (2015), *Deadly Choices. How the Anti-Vaccine Movement Threatens Us All*, New York, Basic Books.

Ogilvie, G. *et al.* (2010), *A Population-Based Evaluation of a Publicly Funded, School-Based HPV Vaccine Program in British Columbia, Canada: Parental Factors Associated With HPV Vaccine Receipt,* "PLoS Med", 7 (5).

O'Leary, S. T., Allison, M. A. *et al.* (2015). *Characteristics of Physicians Who Dismiss Families for Refusing Vaccines,* "Pediatrics", 136(6): 1103–11.

Ołpiński, M. (2012), *Anti-Vaccination Movement and Parental Refusals of Immunization of Children in USA,* "Pediatria Polska", 87(4), pp. 381–85.

Ozawa S., Portnoy A., et al. (2016), *Modeling The Economic Burden Of Adult Vaccine-Preventable Diseases In The United States,* "Health Affairs", 35 (11), pp. 2124–2132.

Panza, F. *et al.* (2014), *Amyloid-Directed Monoclonal Antibodies for the Treatment of Alzheimer's Disease: The Point Of No Return?,* "Expert Opinion on Biological Therapy", 14 (10), pp. 1465–76.

Payet, M. (2017), *Pourquoi ces 200 médecins disent oui aux vaccins obligatoires,* "Le Parisien", 29 June 2017 (https://goo.gl/sFyUvB)

Pead, P. J. (2003), *Benjamin Jesty: new light in the dawn of vaccination,* "Lancet", 362 (9401), 2104–9.

Pegorie, M *et al.* (2014), *Measles Outbreak in Greater Manchester, England, October 2012 to September 2013: Epidemiology and Control,* "Euro Surveill", 18(49).

Peltola, H. *et al.* (1998), *No Evidence for Measles, Mumps, And Rubella Vaccine-Associated Inflammatory Bowel Disease or Autism in A 14-Year Prospective Study,* "Lancet", May 2, 351(9112), pp. 1327, 1328.

Phadke, V. K., *et al.* (2016). *Association Between Vaccine Refusal and Vaccine-Preventable Diseases in the United States: A Review of Measles and Pertussis.* "JAMA" 315(11): 1149–58.

Pierik, R. (2017). *On religious and secular exemptions: A case study of childhood vaccination waivers.* "Ethnicities" 17(2): 220–241.

Pittman, P.R. *et al.* (2004), *Long-Term Health Effects of Repeated Exposure to Multiple Vaccines,* "Vaccine" 23(4), pp. 525–36.

Plett, P. C. (2006), *Peter Plett und die ubrigen Entdecker der Kuhpockenimpfung vor Edward Jenner,* "Sudhoffs Arch", 90 (2), 219–32.

Plotkin, S.A. and S.L. Plotkin (2011), *The Development of Vaccines: How the Past Led to the Future,* "Nature Reviews Microbiology", 9 (12), pp. 889–93.

Poland, G.A. and R. Spier (2010), *Fear, Misinformation, And Innumerates: How The Wakefield Paper, The Press, And Advocacy Groups Damaged The Public Health,* "Vaccine", 28 (12), pp. 2361, 2362.

Porter, D. and Porter R. (1988), *The Politics of Prevention: Anti-Vaccination And Public Health in 19th Century England,* "Medical History", 32, pp. 231–52.

Posfay-Barbe, K.M. *et al.*, *How Do Physicians Immunize Their Own Children? Differences Among Pediatricians and Nonpediatricians,* "Pediatrics", 2005, 116 (5), pp. e623–33.

Pylarini, J. (1716), *A New and Safe Method of Communicating the Small-Pox by Inoculation, Lately Invented and Brought into Us,* in *Philosophical Transactions of the Royal Society of London, from Their Commencement, in 1665, to the Year 1800/ Abridged with Vol. VI from 1713 to 1723*, L & R Baldwin, London.

Ramsingh, A.I. *et al.* (2015), *Transcriptional Dysregulation of Inflammatory/Immune Pathways After Active Vaccination Against Huntington's Disease*, "Human Molecular Genetics".

Rappuoli, R. (2014), *Vaccines: Science, Health, Longevity, And Wealth*, "Proceedings of the National Academy of Sciences of the United States of America", 111 (34), p. 12.282.

Rappuoli, R. and L. Vozza (2009), *I vaccini dell'era globale*, Bologna, Zanichelli.

Reich J.A. (2016), *Calling the shots : why parents reject vaccines*, New York, New York University Press.

Rezza, G. (2010), *Epidemie. Origini ed evoluzione*, Carocci, Roma.

Riedel, S. (2005), *Edward Jenner And the History of Smallpox And Vaccination*, "Proceedings", Baylor University. Medical Center, 18(1), pp. 21–25.

Rieder, M.J. and J.L. Robinson (2015), *Nosodes' Are No Substitute For Vaccines*, "Paediatr Child Health", 20(4), pp. 219–22.

Roehr, B. (2013), *Study Finds No Association Between Vaccines and Autism*, "British Medical Journal", 3 April; 346, p. f2095.

Roggendorf H, Mankertz A, Kundt R, Roggendorf M., Spotlight on measles 2010: measles outbreak in a mainly unvaccinated community in Essen, Germany, March-June 2010. Euro Surveill. 2010 Jul 1;15(26). pii: 19605.

Rook, G.A.W., C.A. Lowry and C.L. Raison (2013), *Microbial "Old Friends", Immunoregulation and Stress Resilience*, "Evolution, Medicine, and Public Health", 2013 (1), pp. 46–64.

Rose, L., M. Browne, et al. (2016). *Scepticism towards vaccination is associated with anti-scientific attitudes and related cultural factors.* "Focus on Alternative and Complementary Therapies" 21(1): 58–59.

Rosenstock, L., & Lee, L. J. (2002). Attacks on Science: The Risks to Evidence-Based Policy. American Journal of Public Health, 92(1), 14–18.

Rota, J. S. *et al.* (2001), *Processes for Obtaining Nonmedical Exemptions to State Immunization Laws*, "American Journal of Public Health", 91(4), p. 645–48.

Ruiz, J.B. e R.A. Bell (2014), *Understanding Vaccination Resistance: Vaccine Search Term Selection Bias and the Valence of Retrieved Information*, "Vaccine", 32 (44), pp. 5776–80.

Ryser, A. J., Heininger U. (2015), *Comparative acceptance of pertussis and influenza immunization among health-care personnel*, "Vaccine", 33 (41), 5350–6.

Salminen, S. *et al.* (2004), *Influence of Mode of Delivery on Gut Microbiota Composition in Seven Year Old Children*, "Gut", 53 (9), pp. 1388, 1389.

Sandin, S. *et al.* (2015), *Autism Risk Associated With Parental Age and With Increasing Difference in Age Between the Parents*, "Molecular Psychiatry", pp. 1–18.

Sandler, B.P. (1941), *The Production of Neuronal Injury And Necrosis With the Virus of Poliomyelitis in Rabbits During Insulin Hypoglycemia* , "The American Journal of Pathology", 17 (1), pp. 69–85.

Schmid, D. *et al.* (2010), *Measles Outbreak Linked to A Minority Group In Austria, 2008*, "Epidemiol Infect", 138 (3), pp. 415–25.

Schmidt, K. and E. Ernst (2002), *Aspects of MMR. Survey Shows that Some Homoeopaths and Chiropractors Advise Against MMR*, "BMJ", 325 (7364), p. 597.

Schmitz, R. *et al.* (2011), *Vaccination Status and Health in Children and Adolescents*, "Dtsch Arztebl International", 108 (7), pp. 99–104.

Schonberger, K. *et al.* (2009), *Risk Factors for Delayed or Missed Measles Vaccination In Young Children*, "Bundesgesundheitsblatt Gesundheitsforschung Gesundheitsschutz", 52 (11), pp. 1045–51.

Shermer, M. (2011), *The real science behind scientology*, "Scientific American" 305(5): 94.

Silvestrini, B. (2014), *Il farmaco moderno: un patto esemplare fra uomo e natura*, Roma, Carocci.

Simpson, N., S. Lenton and R. Randall (1995), *Parental Refusal to Have Children Immunised: Extent And Reasons*. "British Medical Journal", 310 (6974), p. 227.

Singh G. and G. Triadafilopoulos (1999), *Epidemiology of Nsaid Induced Gastrointestinal Complications*, "Journal of Rheumatology Suppl.", 56, pp. 18–24.

Singh, G.K. and M. Siahpush (2014), *Widening Rural-Urban Disparities in All-Cause Mortality and Mortality from Major Causes of Death in the USA, 1969–2009*, "Journal of Urban Health", 91 (2), pp. 272–92.

Smith P.J., Chu S.Y., *et al.*. (2004), *Children Who Have Received No Vaccines: Who Are They and Where Do They Live?*, "Pediatrics", 114 (1), pp. 187–195.

Sobo, E.J. (2015), *Social Cultivation of Vaccine Refusal and Delay among Waldorf (Steiner) School Parents*, "Medical Anthropology Quarterly", 29 (3), pp. 381–399.

Sternhell, Z. (2010). *The anti-enlightenment tradition.* New Haven; London, Yale University Press.

Sun L.H. (2017), *California vaccination rate hits new high after tougher immunization law*, "The Washington Post", April 13th 2017 (https://goo.gl/Nxz1Ai)

Suro, R. (1986) *Italy Acting to End the Sale of Methanol-Tainted Wine*, "The New York Times" April 9th, 1986

Sutton, S. (2008), *Determinants of Health-Related Behaviours: Theoretical and Methodological Issues*, "The SAGE Handbook of Health Psychology", London, pp. 94–127.

Tannous, L.K., G. Barlow e N.H. Metcalfe (2014), *A Short Clinical Review of Vaccination Against Measles*, "JRSM Open", 5 (4).

Tauber, A. I., Podolsky, S. H. (1997). *The generation of diversity: clonal selection theory and the rise of molecular immunology.* Cambridge, Mass., Harvard University Press.

Taylor, B. (2006), *Vaccines and the Changing Epidemiology of Autism*, "Child: Care, Health and Development", 32(5), pp. 511–19.

Taylor, B. *et al.* (1999). *Autism and Measles, Mumps, and Rubella Vaccine: No Epidemiological Evidence For a Causal Association*, "Lancet", June 12, 353(9169), pp. 2026–29.

Tearne, J.E. *et al.* (2015), *Older Maternal Age is Associated With Depression, Anxiety, and Stress Symptoms in Young Adult Female Offspring*, "Journal of Abnormal Psychol", 125 (1), pp. 1–10.

Thaler, R.H. e C.R. Sunstein (2008), *Nudge: Improving Decisions about Health, Wealth, and Happiness.*

Thompson, N.P. *et al.* (1995), *Is Measles Vaccination a Risk Factor for Inflammatory Bowel Disease?*, "Lancet", 345 (8957), pp. 1071–74.

Thurston L, Williams G., An examination of John Fewster's role in the discovery of smallpox vaccination. J R Coll Physicians Edinb. 2015;45(2):173–9.

Til HP, Woutersen RA, Feron VJ, Hollanders VH, Falke HE, Clary JJ. Two-year drinking-water study of formaldehyde in rats. Food Chem Toxicol. 1989 Feb;27 (2):77–87.

Timonius, E. (1714), *An Account, or History, of the Procuring the Small Pox by Incision, or Inoculation; As It Has for Some Time Been Practised at Constantinople*, "Philosophical Transactions of the Royal Society", 29, 338–350, pp. 72–82.

Todd, D. *et al.* (2014), *A Monoclonal Antibody TRKB Receptor Agonist as A Potential Therapeutic for Huntington's Disease*, "PLoS One 9" (2), p. e87.923.

Tucidide, *La guerra del Peloponneso*, edizione con testo greco a fronte, Einaudi, Torino 1996.

Tversky A, Kahneman D., Judgment under Uncertainty: Heuristics and Biases. Science. 1974 Sep 27;185(4157):1124–31.

Uno Y. *et al.* (2015), *Early Exposure to the Combined Measles-Mumps-Rubella Vaccine and Thimerosal-Containing Vaccines and Risk of Autism Spectrum Disorder*, "Vaccine", 33 (21), pp. 2511–16.

Van den Hof, S. *et al.* (2006), *Measles Epidemic in The Netherlands, 1999-2000*, "The Journal of Infectious Diseases", 1876, pp. 1483–86.

Van Der Weyden, M.B., *et al.* (2005), *The 2005 Nobel Prize in Physiology or Medicine*, "Medical Journal of Australia", 183 (11–12), pp. 612–14.

Van Velzen, E. *et al.* (2008), *Measles Outbreak in An Anthroposophic Community in The Hague, The Netherlands, June-July*, "Euro Surveill", 13, p. 31.

Verstraeten T. *et al.* (2003), *Safety of Thimerosal-Containing Vaccines: A Two-Phased Study of Computerized Health Maintenance Organization Databases*, "Pediatrics", 112 (5), pp. 1039–48.

Vesikari T. *et al.* (2011*), Oil-In-Water Emulsion Adjuvant with Influenza Vaccine in Young Children*, "The New England Journal of Medicine", 365 (15), pp. 1406–16.

Viscusi, W.K. (1997). *Alarmist Decisions With Divergent Risk Information*, "Economic Journal", 107(445), pp. 1657–70.

Vivancos, R. *et al.* (2012), *An Ongoing Large Outbreak of Measles in Merseyside, England, January to June 2012*, "Euro Surveill", 17(29).

Vozza, L., D'Incalci, M., & Gescher, A. (2017). How medicines are born: The imperfect science of drugs. London, Hackensack, NJ : World Scientific Publishing Europe Ltd.

Wakefield, A.J. (2003), *Measles, Mumps, and Rubella Vaccination and Autism. Comment to the* Editor, "The New England Journal of Medicine", 348 (10), p. 952.

Wakefield A.J. *et al.* (1993), *Evidence of Persistent Measles Virus Infection in Crohn's Disease,* "Journal of Medical Virology", 39 (4), pp. 345–53.

Wakefield, A.J. *et al.* (1998), *Ileal-Lymphoid-Nodular Hyperplasia, Non-Specific Colitis, and Pervasive Developmental Disorder in Children,* "Lancet", 351 (9103), pp. 637–41.

Walkinshaw, E. (2011), *Mandatory Vaccinations: The International Landscape,* "Canadian Medical Association Journal", 183(16), pp. e1167, e1168.

Watier, H. (2009), *From the Ancient Serotherapy to Naked Antibodies: A Century of Successful Targeted Therapie*s, "Médecine/Sciences" (Paris), 25(12), pp. 999–1009.

WHO (2009), *Measles Vaccines: WHO Position Paper,* "Weekly Epidemiological Record", N. 35. 84, 349–60.

Wicker, S. , Rose, M. A. (2011), *Health care workers and pertussis: an underestimated issue,* "Med Klin" (Munich), 105 (12), 882–6.

Williamson, P. (2016), *Take the time and effort to correct misinformation,* "Nature", 540(7632), Dec.,171–171.

Wolfe, N.D., C.P. Dunavan and J. Diamond (2007), *Origins of Major Human Infectious Diseases,* "Nature", 447 (7142), pp. 279–83.

Wolfe, R.M. and L.K. Sharp (2002), *Anti-Vaccinationists Past and Present,* "British Medical Journal", 325, pp. 430–32.

Wood, M.J., K.M. Douglas and R.M. Sutton (2012), *Dead and Alive: Beliefs in Contradictory Conspiracy Theories,* "Social Psychological and Personality Science", 3 (6), pp. 767–73.

Xie, S. and D. Zhang (2000), *Spread of Chinese Variolation Art to The Western World and Its Influence,* "Zhonghua Yi Shi Za Zhi", 30(3), pp. 133–37.

Xin-Zhong, Y. (2003*), A Preliminary Study of Vaccination in Jiangnan During the Qing Dynasty,* "Studies in Qing History", 2, pp. 28–37.

Yaqub O., Castle-Clarke S. et al. (2014), *Attitudes to vaccination: A critical review,* "Social Science & Medicine", 112, pp. 1–11.

Yih, W.K., E. Weintraub and M. Kulldorff (2012), *No Risk of Guillain-Barre Syndrome Found After Meningococcal Conjugate Vaccination in Two Large Cohort Studies,* "Pharmacoepidemiology Drug Safety", 21 (12), pp. 1359–60.

Yong, J. *et al.* (2011), *BCG Vaccine-Induced Neuroprotection in A Mouse Model of Parkinson's Disease,* "PLoS One", 6 (1), p. e16.610.

Young A., Chaudhry H. *et al..* (2015), *A Census of Actively Licensed Physicians in the United States, 2014,* "Journal of Medical Regulation", 101 (2), pp. 8–23.

Young, K. *et al.* (2002), *Social Science and The Evidence-Based Policy Movement,* "Social Policy & Society", Vol.1, N. 3, pp. 215–24.

Zhang J, While AE, Norman IJ, Nurses' knowledge and risk perception towards seasonal influenza and vaccination and their vaccination behaviours: a cross-sectional survey. Int J Nurs Stud. 2011 Oct;48(10):1281–9.

Zhu, J.L. *et al.* (2008), *Paternal Age and Mortality in Children,* "European Journal Epidemiology", 23 (7), pp. 443–47.

Zoja L. (2011), *Paranoia: la follia che fa la storia*. Torino, Bollati Boringhieri (English translation: *Paranoia The madness that makes history*. Florence, Taylor and Francis, 2017).

Zollo, F. *et al.* (2015), *Debunking in a World of Tribes*, (in press) available in preprint arXiv:1510.04267.

Zuzak, T.J. *et al.* (2008), *Attitudes Towards Vaccination: Users of Complementary and Alternative Medicine Versus Non-Users*, "Swiss Medical Weekly", 138 (47–48), pp. 713–18.

Printed in the United States
By Bookmasters